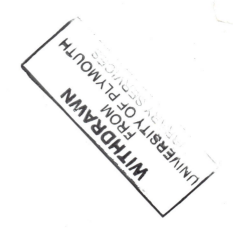
Neil MacKay

REMOVING DYSLEXIA AS A BARRIER TO ACHIEVEMENT

The Dyslexia Friendly Schools Toolkit

SEN Marketing

www.senbooks.co.uk

COPYRIGHT STATEMENT

Copyright © SEN Marketing
618 Leeds Road, Outwood
Wakefield   WF1 2LT
Tel: 01924 871697
www.senbooks.co.uk

ISBN 1 903842 05 0

2nd Edition, September 2006
First published, June 2005

Dedication

This book is dedicated to my family, Carole, Jamie, Beth and Corinne with grateful thanks for their love and support.

Also to the staff, pupils and parents of Hawarden High School who taught me so much.

REMOVING DYSLEXIA AS A BARRIER TO ACHIEVEMENT

The Dyslexia Friendly Schools Toolkit

Contents

FOREWORD

I am pleased to provide an introduction to 'Removing Dyslexia as a Barrier to Achievement' since it endorses and provides comprehensive advice on how all lessons for all learners are planned, resourced and taught in school.

In this way it brings to our attention the issue of providing the best opportunities for each of the learners in the mainstream classroom, whatever their learning difference or style - a very important point to address since this represents, for the most part, where the majority of dyslexic learners spend most of their time.

Neil MacKay's book takes a thought provoking and detailed look at the potential to create Dyslexia Friendly learning environments – in the classroom and the school and as such his book is very much in line with the British Dyslexia Association's initiative - 'Inclusive Education : Dyslexia Friendly Quality Mark for Children's Services and Schools'.

The Dyslexia Friendly Toolkit is full of practical guidance, empowering ideas and challenging assertions about inclusion. It presents many strategies for meeting diverse learning needs, and methods for overcoming barriers to learning. These are clearly rooted in practice and based on a wealth of relevant experience that the author has deftly woven into the narrative.

Removing Dyslexia as a Barrier to Achievement has the potential to make a valuable contribution to enabling dyslexic learners, and indeed all learners with their varied learning styles, to fulfil their potential and realise their learning aspirations.

Professor Susan Tresman
Chief Executive
British Dyslexia Association

June 2005.

Chapter 1

DYSLEXIA – DIFFICULTY OR DIFFERENCE?

The accepted view of Dyslexia as a specific learning difficulty may have been a major cause of under achievement among learners and low expectations among teachers for the past two or three decades. A learning difficulty implies that something is "wrong" with the learner, leading to a focus on identifying weaknesses rather than celebrating strengths. This, in turn, can result in an emphasis on remediation by specialists rather than resolution by aware class and subject teachers through reasonable adjustments. One inevitable consequence of this has been to focus on a school's special needs provision, placing responsibility for remediation on the SENCO and diverting attention away from Quality First teaching in the mainstream classroom which is, after all, the place where dyslexic learners spend most of their time.

Acknowledging, SpLD as a Specific Learning Difference, places the focus firmly on how all lessons are planned, resourced and taught, and also on the way teachers are supported through the school policy, practice and ethos. This position offers real opportunities for an emphasis on inclusive mainstream strategies which are designed to empower all learners to be the best they can be. For the purpose of this book, therefore, Dyslexia will be defined as:

> *"A specific learning difference for any given level of ability, which may cause unexpected difficulties, in the acquisition of certain skills"*

This definition is deliberately short, simple and straightforward. Many current definitions are little more than descriptions and so full of exceptions, caveats and sub clauses that they are positively dyslexia unfriendly and make little sense to busy practitioners in the classroom; I would also question their relevance to parents and children. This definition has been presented to thousands of mainstream teachers and it seems to strike a chord – you can actually see them running their eye over the learners in the class and mentally ticking off those with this learning difference. It also establishes Dyslexia as an issue at all levels of ability and arguably as a learning preference.

Defining Dyslexia as a specific learning difference, rather than a difficulty, conveys a realistic balance of opportunities and costs, and strengths and weaknesses for the child, as do all the other learning styles and preferences. The "straight line thinking" typical of many mathematical logical learners is vulnerable when creativity is required, while the eclectic style of linguistic learners may not yield results when the task calls for step by step processing. So, while continuing to acknowledge that some dyslexic learners will require discrete specialist support at some time, the notion of Dyslexia as a specific learning difficulty is arguably unhelpful and wrong, certainly within the inclusive ethos of a Dyslexia Friendly classroom.

While there are undoubted areas of vulnerability, this is true of all learners and of all learning preferences.   The skill of the teacher lies in achieving a balance between empowerment and challenge within clearly understood patterns of strength and weakness. Therefore, viewing Dyslexia as a difficulty may be to misunderstand the situation. In the mainstream classroom, dyslexia is, in fact, a specific learning difference which becomes a difficulty when ignored, dismissed or badly addressed.

How does this difference manifest?

Dyslexic learners are often imaginative and creative lateral thinkers who develop original solutions to problems.   They may be skilful in design and construction, IT etc, often seeming to "know" how things work without reading instructions, manuals etc.

One specific learning difference may be the ability to "think in pictures," sometimes with original artistic talent and often with a strong visual preference in terms of information acquisition and processing. Some dyslexic children and adults seem to be able run a test programme or sequence through in their mind in "video" and actually visualise what will happen when elements or parameters are changed.   Many dyslexic learners are sociable and verbally able and may enjoy drama and sport. Typically they will demonstrate ability appropriate interest in science, technology or current affairs, often with a general knowledge to match.

Dyslexia is:

"A specific learning difference which, at any level of ability, may cause unexpected difficulties in the acquisition of certain skills"

The specific difference enables some learners to be curious, eclectic and creative, identifying links and patterns unclear to others. Creating a big picture from apparently disparate bits is often a strength, as is the ability to form the "whole", when some of the elements are missing or not quite appropriate. However it is essential to keep in mind that these various strengths need to be benchmarked against other learners of the same ability.

Despite opportunities there are inevitable costs associated with thinking in a dyslexic way, just as there are with all the other learning styles and preferences. The nature of the specific learning difference may cause unexpected problems with the acquisition of basic literacy and numeracy skills, requiring dyslexic children to be taught in the way they learn in order to minimize problems and maximize potential. A particular priority is to recognize and compensate for possible problems with working memory, information processing and hearing the sounds and syllables in words.

Dyslexic learners are particularly vulnerable when a classroom-based preoccupation with reading and spelling accuracy is allowed to detract from information processing and organizing thoughts on paper. When this happens the specific difference becomes a specific difficulty and a learning preference becomes a learning problem. Placing undue emphasis on accurate reading, writing, spelling and number as an end product rather than as a process is unhelpful, if not harmful. This is not to deny the importance of quality intervention to develop and improve skill levels in areas of weakness. However this is the right of all learners – a basic entitlement to whatever is required in order for them to access the curriculum at an ability appropriate level.

Moving towards the difference

More and more schools, with the active and enthusiastic support of their Children's Services, are aspiring to become Dyslexia Friendly. The ideas and challenges launched by the BDA Dyslexia Friendly Schools packs are striking a chord across the UK and beyond as teachers begin to realise that the fine tuning needed to make schools Dyslexia Friendly has the potential to improve the learning of all pupils. It needs to be clearly stated however, that this initiative is not about special educational needs, nor is it necessarily the domain of Special Needs Coordinators (SENCOs) unless they are already members of the school's senior management team. Becoming a Dyslexia Friendly school requires a review of the implementation of major whole school policies, especially teaching and learning, monitoring and assessment, differentiation and inclusion. The issue then becomes one of how these policies are monitored, evaluated and reviewed to ensure top quality learning right across the range of ability and need – a Dyslexia Friendly school enhances the learning of all.

The DYSLEXIA FRIENDLY SCHOOLS Initiative

- Teaching mainstream classes which contain dyslexic learners

- Inclusion through good classroom practice

- Monitoring, evaluation and review of the effectiveness of whole school policies to include:

1. Teaching and Learning
2. Monitoring and Assessment
3. Differentiation
4. Parents as Partners

The School that I'd like

Imagine a school which acknowledges that all children learn in different ways and in which teachers harness the power of learning styles and preferences to optimise teaching and learning. In this school teachers also recognise that many apparent learning difficulties can often be explained as learning differences which will respond to changes in methods, materials and approaches. Also many of the special educational needs which formerly occupied the attention of class/subject teachers and SENCOs may now be seen as ordinary learning needs which are dealt with in mainstream settings through the differentiated curriculum plan. As a result the school is writing far fewer Individual Education Plans (IEPs): those that are written are of high quality, and are very carefully monitored and evaluated to actively direct and inform the way children are taught in mainstream settings.

This school is particularly aware of the needs of the growing numbers of non-traditional learners who do not function well in a didactic environment and who often think faster than they read, write, spell or do number work. Therefore there is a house style, evident in every classroom, in which children are required to explore ideas, concepts and strategies within the framework of their preferred learning styles. They are also actively encouraged to present evidence of their learning and understanding within these styles.

An interesting aspect of this school is the calm, confident way in which all children approach their learning. Even the most vulnerable learners are set up to succeed because they are effectively working within their comfort zones for much of the time and operating from a secure platform of strength and competence. When challenged to move outside their comfort zones they are able to respond with confidence because of their platform of previous success. One consequence of this confidence and emotional security is the positive way in which all children approach assessments, even some of those national assessments which seem to be carefully engineered to marginalise children who learn in non-traditional ways. Although this school is very successful in terms of results, it values this success less than it values it's eclectic, confident and independent learners who are developing across the full range of ability and social, emotional and intellectual need.

This school is Dyslexia Friendly, without a doubt. However it is also learning friendly, seeking to empower all pupils to be the best they can be. That is the incentive for becoming a Dyslexia Friendly school.

The advantages are significant, with a positive "opportunity cost". However it must be understood that the implementation of whole school change needs to be the responsibility of someone who has the position, authority and support to drive the cycles of implementation, evaluation and review.

Perhaps it all hinges on the way ability or intelligence is viewed. For the purpose of this book, intelligence is defined as:

"Knowing what to do when you don't know what to do".

By this definition, an intelligent learner has an internal conversation which goes something like, "What I'm doing isn't working and I don't really know what to do here, so what I'll do is..." Yet there is still a residual belief among parents, politicians and some teachers and inspectors that the measure of intelligence is accurate reading, writing, spelling and number. While it is fair to say that more and more teachers are recognising that weak basic skills bear little relationship to ability and intelligence, this message seems to be slow to filter up to the policy shapers, as evidenced by current assessment strategies and curricular reforms. Teachers who believe that thinking and conceptual development are key measures of intelligence and who find creative ways to empower pupils to show what they know in a variety of ways are naturally Dyslexia Friendly because they are "learning friendly". They focus on strengths and use these strengths to address the unexpected problems that dyslexic learners seem to experience in certain areas.

The "unexpected" problems tend to arise in the acquisition and application of aspects of basic skills. These problems often occur despite adequate opportunity to learn and are highlighted against a background of ability appropriate skill acquisition in other areas. Dyslexic learners are usually as good as their peers at many things and are fine until, for example, they need to write it down.   In the mainstream classroom where dyslexic learners spend most, if not all of their time, problems seem to occur in four main areas:

The School that I'd Like?

Run by idealists with a strategy

- Dyslexia Friendly = Mind Friendly

- Celebrating learning difference

- Recognising learning preferences

- Accepting work in different forms

- Developing emotional literacy

1. Visual sequential working memory – remembering what you see, in the order in which you see it, long enough to do something with the information. Weaknesses in this area contribute to issues like poor reading accuracy and identifying spelling errors.

2. Auditory sequential working memory – remembering what you hear, in the order in which you hear it and being able to hold it long enough to make an appropriate response. Following instructions may be a challenge, as will chunking complex words into syllables in order to decode them.

3. Information processing – the ability to process information and present it in an appropriate form. This information may need to be remembered from recent instruction or retrieved from previous knowledge and then selected and ordered to perform a task. Using a climate graph to write a holiday postcard about the weather requires information processing to select, order and present graphical information in narrative form.

4. Phonological awareness – being able to hear sounds in words and to associate the sounds with appropriate letter combinations. Implicit within this is the ability to break down and re-build words. Spelling and/or reading complex jargon words are often challenges for dyslexic learners, but if they can clap the rhythm and "stretch" the word, the parts become clearer and can often be written in a way which, if not correct, is close enough not to be a barrier to communication.

These four aspects may be considered to be largely "intelligence free" - most learners develop the skills at an ability appropriate level as the result of appropriate teaching and learning. The concept of "ability appropriate" is the key to an understanding of this issue.

A Specific Learning Difference

creating

"Unexpected Difficulties in relation to Ability":

- **Auditory sequential memory**

- **Visual sequential memory**

- **Information processing**

- **Phonological Awareness**

Unexpected Difficulties in relation to ability?

Consider the performance of two children, both of whom have average verbal and non-verbal reasoning skills. One child has ability appropriate skills in reading accuracy/comprehension and spelling – the other does not, despite apparently having the ability to do so and is experiencing unexpected problems in developing ability appropriate basic skills. Consequently there are few intellectual barriers to prevent the child from performing at an ability appropriate level in all aspects of work that do not involve reading, writing or spelling. However specific difficulties may kick in and significantly depress performance if the learner is not taught in the ways s/he prefers to learn. Also, at this point in the lesson, the baggage from years of difficulties in these areas may also manifest in the form of lack of self belief, low self esteem and poor motivation.

Arguably emotional strength and confidence are the keys to maximising strengths and minimising weaknesses. These emotional issues can compound the weakness unless addressed through effective classroom management, quality pupil teacher relationships and appropriately differentiated tasks delivered in a high challenge, low stress environment. Unfortunately, conceptual abilities that do not translate into written or "mark-able" work may be undervalued or even ignored in major assessments. This is certainly the case in national tests conducted in the UK at ages 7, 10, 14 and 16 and may explain why many dyslexic learners seem to come into their own later in life, when they can pick their way through further and higher education in ways which suit their learning styles and preferences.

> # The key to maximising strengths and minimising weaknesses?
>
> # Emotional strength and Confidence

Summary

- Dyslexia is a specific learning difference

- It becomes a difficulty when different learning needs are ignored or marginalised

- A learner with weak basic skills, who can understand, think, argue and create at an ability appropriate level may have a specific learning difference if positive answers are given to the following questions:

    1. Has s/he had adequate opportunity to develop basic skills?

    2. Is the basic skills issue unexpected in the light of other strengths?

    3. Have other pupils at the same level of ability and with apparently similar problems made progress with the same level/style of teaching?

- If the answer is "yes" to all three, then it is possible that the child has a specific learning difference which, if not facilitated, will quickly turn into a specific learning difficulty

16

DIFFERENCE

OR

DIFFICULTY?

Schools and teachers have the power to decide:

"Schools should not assume that children's difficulties always result solely, or even mainly, from problems within the child. A school's practices make a difference, for good or evil."

(DfES SEN Code of Practice)

Chapter 2

UNDERSTANDING DYSLEXIA – REMOVING BARRIERS

This section will look at the way Dyslexia may manifest in the classroom and the important questions - "What do I look out for?" and "What do I do if and when I think Dyslexia might be an issue?" It is not the purpose of this section to label a child as dyslexic. Rather it is to support teachers to identify those learners who will benefit from Dyslexia Friendly approaches, and to develop "dyslexia antennae".

Family History

It is generally accepted that Dyslexia often runs in families; having parents who are dyslexic significantly increases the incidence. It is also common for someone in the wider family to be dyslexic, rather than just parents, and the condition can also occur without any familial incidence. Considerable time, energy and funding continues to be devoted to identifying the "dyslexic gene" presumably with a view to developing gene therapy to eliminate it. This is to miss the fundamental point that Dyslexia can be a valuable learning difference that conveys real gifts and the "right to be dyslexic" is fundamental. Many difficulties are, as acknowledged in the UK Code of Practice, often the result of school-based problems relating to an obsession with literacy targets, poor resourcing and a focus on teaching rather than learning.

However, in successful schools dyslexic learners are being taught how to build on their strengths, minimise their weaknesses and are empowered to be the best they can be. Therefore a re-focussing of research funding into the classroom implications of Dyslexia as a learning difference will prove to be very inclusive, effective and beneficial. Future researchers would perhaps do well to recognise that the solution to the Dyslexia issue lies primarily with providing support strategies which work in mainstream classrooms, strategies which can be delivered by very busy, often non specialist teachers who are required to meet the needs of dyslexic learners alongside the needs of every child in the class.

When a parent suggests that a child is dyslexic it is always worth asking if anyone in the wider family has a similar pattern of strengths and weaknesses. If parents are not dyslexic, there will often be uncles, aunts and/or cousins who have perhaps successfully channelled their energy and ability into jobs less reliant on accurate basic skills. Unfortunately there will be others who have been damaged by the system and who have profoundly under-achieved. During this initial conversation it is also helpful to encourage parents to consider their child's strengths.

Anxious parents understandably focus on problems, but finding out that the child may have very strong IT skills, is good at making/mending, perhaps talented at drama or art, or has great general knowledge, all help to benchmark current basic skill weaknesses within a framework of the other strengths and abilities which represent this child's learning differences.

Early to walk – may not crawl

Research using MRI technology is showing that the brain of a dyslexic child or adult is differently "wired": there is a different pattern of activity in the brain that may account for a learning difference. Consequently Dyslexia appears to be a neurological "given". The subject is dyslexic, will always be so and will have a wide range of learning preferences just like the rest of the population. Therefore it is up to all individuals to make best use of the pattern of strengths and weaknesses conferred by their brain organisation. There is also a growing understanding of the link between motor development and the acquisition of some basic skills. Activities that improve coordination, like Brain Gym, seem to integrate the cerebellum and promote the acquisition of basic skills in some children. Some dyslexic children seem to miss the crawling stage, going straight from "bottom shuffling" to walking. It has been reported that non-reading adults have learnt to read following a course of crawling activities; so asking about crawling may help to build a picture.

Dressing skills

Unexpected problems with the acquisition of dressing skills are also commonly reported. This is why nursery nurses are often the first people to recognise and respond to early signs of Dyslexia. Consider a child whose brothers and/or sisters have already passed through the nursery. These siblings all had age/ability appropriate dressing skills, implying that they had been taught as part of the normal parenting process. This child, however, cannot manage some aspects of dressing or perhaps does not seem to appreciate the order that clothes need to be put on. This is unexpected, because s/he has clearly been taught the skills in the same way as the siblings, and so it becomes another indicator of a learning difference. The significance of this indicator is compounded if the child is found to have other coordinational strengths, perhaps with Lego, Sticklebricks, or wiring simple circuits etc.

Labels, rhymes and sequences

These are an aspect of many tests for Dyslexia, but testing is not the only way to identify specific learning differences or any resulting difficulties. Issues to do with sequential memory, word finding or rhyming are quickly and easily identifiable in the classroom, without necessarily resorting to testing. What must be avoided, at all costs, is the refrain, "We think s/he is dyslexic but we are waiting for the Psychologist to do an assessment before we can do anything." This response is the typical and flawed "SEN" approach which requires learners to fail, often for protracted periods of time, in order to become eligible for intervention. Indeed, in a worst case scenario, learners have to fail for weeks and months before they can even be considered for intervention, let alone receive any.

One advantage of a pragmatic identification of issues is that an immediate, classroom-based response can be made (rather than going through a process of referral for testing) with the teacher making reasonable adjustments as a part of a commitment to Quality First teaching. The result of this intervention will determine the need for further action. If it works, the root cause is probably a lack of opportunity to develop the skills, something which early years teachers report as being increasingly common. If intervention does not work then this may indicate that something a bit more "special" is required in terms of strategies and programmes of support. Children for whom English is an additional language may also be vulnerable in terms of labels, rhymes and sequences, their problems decreasing as their language skills develop.

When a child fails to develop, when others with apparently similar needs begin to do so, and especially when there are clear strengths in other areas, then we are probably looking at the "unexpected" once again.

In the 1980s, Bradley and Bryant observed that young children who could not orally segment words would later experience problems acquiring ability appropriate literacy skills. They adopted a wonderfully pragmatic approach, advocating immediate intervention, without recourse to testing. Their reasoning, quite rightly, was that this would probably resolve the issues for many children. Those who failed to respond quickly probably had more severe and specific issues that needed further intervention. However, little was lost by the pragmatic response which effectively helped individual children without recourse to giving individual help, an effective approach that was also an efficient use of time and resources. The optimum approach for the class teacher is best summed up as "rigorous scrutiny, followed by immediate intervention".

Spells/reads a word on one line, but not on the next

This is a tendency that infuriates teachers and parents and frustrates pupils, especially when learners are accused of laziness and/or lack of concentration. In fact this tendency could be considered to be a key indicator of unexpected difficulties. The problem seems to occur as a result of two key areas of vulnerability for dyslexic learners, their auditory and visual sequential memories. Both memories have limited working space and are easily overloaded, particularly when a learner is stressed and especially during those well-documented "dyslexic days" when little seems to go right. In consequence, a word that has been successfully read/spelt further up the page is completely "new" and unfamiliar the next time it is encountered. Best advice is to treat it as a "can't do it" rather than as a "won't" and respect the learner's difficulty.

Few caring teachers would criticise children with cerebral palsy for being challenged by aspects of motor coordination, yet dyslexic learners are regularly taken to task for something which is equally beyond their control. Dyslexia Friendly teachers recognise that the problem word is effectively a new word for the learner at this time, regardless of successful reading/spelling at another time, and adopt an empathic approach which minimises stress, maximises ability and pays due attention to the learner's vulnerable self-image.

Quick thinker/doer, but not necessarily when given instructions

Dyslexic learners are often very quick to make connections and to solve problems, but not always when given instructions. The differently wired brain sometimes slows down the processes associated with receptive language and can inhibit rapid/automatic responses to instructions and/or questions – mental maths and other "quick fire" challenges can often leave the learner exposed and frustrated.

When "take up time" is given dyslexic learners can function as well, if not better than others of similar ability. A failure to achieve automaticity in certain key tasks may be regarded as a positive indicator of dyslexia and may manifest in things like multiplication tables, number bonds, alphabetical sequencing, referencing and spelling.

When given time to reflect, dyslexic learners often produce answers that are as good, if not better, than their faster reacting peers. There can be a tendency to perceive a quick response as a sign of intelligence, whereas in reality a first response may be ill considered or even wrong. The reflective quality of dyslexic learners' responses may often be of higher quality yet somehow dismissed because of the delay between stimulus and response.

It is interesting to contrast the way question and answer sessions are conducted in the UK and in Japan. In the UK children raise their hands and are often very vocal in their attempts to attract the teacher's attention. As a result it takes a strong teacher to ignore the forest of hands and to encourage reflective thinkers to provide a fair share of the answers. In Japan, however, children often only answer when asked to respond. This cultural difference would seem to empower reflective thinkers to involve themselves without the pressure of having to be first in order to be acknowledged.

Dyslexic Difficulties?

More often a "can't do"

Rather than a "won't do"

So

"Accentuate the Positive"

Enhanced creativity

Not all dyslexic learners are creative, but those who are, will often be very original thinkers who consistently come up with unique solutions to problems. The differently wired brain seems to convey the gift of creativity in certain areas, something that is beginning to be recognised by employers.

Careers like architecture; engineering; plastic surgery; art; design; computer graphics; landscape gardening; tree surgery; window dressing and photography are all areas where dyslexic learners seem to excel because they require an ability to see the whole picture, even when bits are currently missing.

When the film "The Titanic" was produced, it had some of the most complex computer generated graphics ever achieved and it is reported that many of the team responsible for this were dyslexic. As the trend develops, carried forward by films like Matrix; Lord of the Rings; X Men, etc, it is likely that there will be active recruitment of dyslexic IT specialists to take the process to higher and higher levels.

This creativity is often evident in the classroom as well. It was Simeon who, when asked to build a hut for his desert island, produced one with running water! He took his steam engine apart, using the piston and cylinder to pump water from a small reservoir. So Simeon's hut had a washbasin with a pumped supply of water.

Aptitude for constructional/technical toys

Who brings in amazing working models, built without recourse to manual or instructions? Who has an intuitive ability to make new software work or to make old programmes operate to their optimum? Who has turned an interest in media into an ability to light a stage so that it actually becomes the real world, bridging reality and theatre in an uncanny way?

So often it is the dyslexic learner who just seems to "know" how it works. This is a rare talent and one which needs celebrating and also to be placed in a proper context against current weaknesses in the acquisition of some basic skills.

> # Success comes in "cans", not "can'ts"
>
> # So
>
> # Give them more of what they are good at
>
> # and
>
> # "Catch them doing it right!"

Appears bright but is an enigma

A picture has been painted of a learner who, like all others in a classroom, is a complex blend of strengths and weaknesses. Dyslexic learners can be enigmas because their skills and talents do not always transfer to some school based tasks. This lack of transfer is particularly evident when a learner gives a competent performance during oral, problem solving tasks and then fails to present written work at the same level. As Howard Gardiner observes, "There is something wrong when a person is able to do some things very well but is not considered smart if these things are not connected with school success". Part of the challenge for teachers is to discover ways of empowering dyslexic learners to feel good about themselves and their abilities.

Summary

Indicators of the need for a Dyslexia Friendly approach include:

- Family history
- Early to walk – perhaps without crawling
- Unexpected difficulties acquiring some dressing skills
- Unexpected difficulties with labels, rhymes and sequences
- Spelling/reading a word on one line but not the next
- Often quick to think and do when it is their choice of task – often much slower to respond to set tasks
- Enhanced creativity
- Aptitude for constructional and technical toys
- A failure to produce written evidence of learning which matches their abilities and skills in other areas

"There is something wrong when a person is able to do some things very well...

but is not considered smart if these things are not connected with school success"

Howard Gardiner

Chapter 3

CREATING THE FEEL-GOOD FACTOR

Supporting learners to feel good about themselves and to appreciate their pattern of strengths and weaknesses is a building block of effective classroom management. The first element for consideration is the attitude of the learners to themselves: secure, happy learners learn - stressed, anxious learners do not.

It is helpful to begin with a breakdown of issues and possible responses. Then it will be necessary to examine some mainstream strategies to support dyslexic learners to be the best they can be within a framework of strengths and weaknesses. A key responsibility of the Dyslexia Friendly teacher is to provide emotional support for vulnerable learners, because it has been suggested that up to 80% of learning difficulties have been attributed to stress. So eliminating classroom stress can minimise the difficulty. Stress may be caused by fear of:

    i.   The teacher's disapproval/lack of understanding
    ii. Failure- in particular the "baggage" from previous failure or the expectation of imminent failure or future failure
    iii. Tests – especially spelling and tables tests
    iv. Reading out loud
    v. Being shouted at

1. Minimising the fear of disapproval/lack of understanding

- Let the child know we understand/appreciate the problem(s)
- Communicate that "It's ok to be dyslexic"
- Make sure our body language and tone communicate the right message
- Use the language of possibility
- Demonstrate our understanding through the consistent use of effective strategies
- Mark for success – ticking words spelt correctly, tick the number of correct letters in a word etc

I would argue that it is inappropriate and unprofessional to tell a child that s/he is dyslexic when a formal assessment has not taken place. However, I can see no problems with talking to children about their specific learning differences, about the ways these differences affect their learning and how to maximise the opportunities and minimise the problems conferred by learning preferences. So it is ok to be a strongly kinaesthetic and visual learner, especially when the Dyslexia Friendly teacher actively promotes situations in which these preferences come to the fore. It is also ok to prefer to access information in ways other than reading and to present information in forms other than sentences and paragraphs. Listening to the voice of the pupil is also extremely helpful, two out of three children need a good listening to!

If the teacher in a Dyslexia Friendly school is required, by policy and ethos, to create opportunities to work within preferences and to develop competencies in weaker, more vulnerable areas then so much the better. Never forget that while good teachers usually reach 80% of pupils in a lesson, great teachers probably reach a different 80% each time! They do this by auditing the learning styles used and ensuring that all preferences are catered for.

As much as 80% of the message we communicate to our learners seems to be in our posture and tone. An open body posture, a welcoming smile that is in our voice and eyes as well as in the words, the way we respond to issues all convey subtle messages to our pupils. Responding to a raised hand with a smile and a "Hi, how can I help?" emphasise that asking for help is expected and welcomed. Using the language of possibility and success is also of key importance. A learner may wail that s/he "can't read/can't spell". The temptation to indulge in a homily about "You can if you try harder" – carries its own implicit put down, especially when maximum effort is actually being made. A more learner friendly response is to do a reality check – point out that while s/he can read and spell lots of words, some will obviously cause problems from time to time.

The Feel-good Factor - 1

80% of Learning Difficulties could be due to stress

Removing the stress leaves 20% of the problem

We can work with that!

2. Minimising a fear of failure

- Use the language of success
- Create "nice one" awards
- Create "error free" learning situations while confidence develops
- Set achievable targets for test scores
- Stress that: "Mistakes are cool because they mean that somebody tried"
- Stress that: "There is no failure, only feedback"
- Avoid: "Death by deep marking"

Of all the words that can convey hope and faith in a learner, "yet" is one of the most powerful. It also communicates empathy and a willingness to share the load. A Dyslexia Friendly response to "I can't do it" could be *"Perhaps you can't do part of it yet. Try this…"* Acknowledging current difficulties in a positive way is equally effective. Phrases like "It *is* a bit tricky – are there any bits I can help you with?" encourage the learner to reflect and share; a question like, "Which bits can I help you with?" is a more assertive alternative.

Both pay the learner the compliment of assuming that some aspects of the task are going well. Less is often more when working with dyslexic learner; just knowing that the teacher is there for them, in a supportive and non-judgemental way, seems to empower some learners to go forward on their own and work it out for themselves. This is rarely the case when encouraged to "try harder". Suggesting that "You can do it if you try" is a put down, since it assumes s/he is not trying already. The positive approach also recognises that, although learners may be stuck at this moment, they may be determined to work it out alone. As a general principle I try never to assume that help is welcome, preferring to offer it with phrases like *"May I help you?"* or *"Would it help if I…"* The decision to accept help should, I believe, always lie with the learner.

The Feel-good Factor – 2

When responding to questions or requests for help and guidance

SMILE before answering

Project the message, "It's ok to ask – I'm glad you did"

A safe classroom is one in which learners can count on their teacher to access tasks effectively and with all due regard to self-image and self-esteem. In a safe class, "mistakes are cool" because they mean that someone has tried. Unconditional acceptance of a learner's finished product is important, especially in the early stages of a relationship. Although the work may actually disappoint both parties, it may represent all that was achievable at that time, especially if the learner is experiencing a "dyslexic day". These are days when life, the universe and everything seem to conspire to reduce a learner's efficiency and make learning a real challenge. Accepting work at face value and involving the learner in the marking and feedback is supportive in this situation. The following questions may be helpful:

- *Which bits do you like/are you happy with?*
  (Note the positive start)
- *Do any bits disappoint you?*
- *Which bits do you think I will be pleased with?*
- *Which bits do you think I will be worried about?*
  (This is a particularly good question. It allows the teacher to demonstrate acceptance and respect by dismissing some or most of the issues identified by the learner)
- *What would you change if you did it again?*
- *What mark/comment would you give yourself?*
  (Another good question, as learners will often be very hard on themselves, allowing the teacher to disagree and boost them up. *"I'm sorry, I can't possibly agree with you. This is worth much more because..."*)
- *Would it help if I gave you a sentence to get you started?*
- *Would it help if we did a quick bit of planning together?*
- *If you don't mind, let's leave this now and go on to the next bit*

The consistent use of these responses reinforces the important message that there is no failure, only feedback and learning. It does cost a little more in terms of time, especially in the early confidence-building stages. The opportunity cost, however, is an increasingly confident and independent learner who will produce better work and require less and less support as the year progresses. I would say that all strategies to improve confidence and capability are a valuable and cost effective investment of time.

Paradoxically, it can be helpful to agree with the learner that it was a poor piece of work and then dismiss it with a comment like *"No problem. It was a bit tricky and you had a good go at it. What I'd like you to do next is…"* The message here is that nobody can be perfect all of the time! Learners who get hung up on success may find themselves paralysed by a fear of failure – dyslexic learners are particularly vulnerable here – and come to realise that, if they do not join the race, they cannot come last.

Choosing when to do an "ok" job and save some energy for when it really counts is important, especially when currently weak basic skills are causing problems. Part of the skill of the teacher, then, is to develop this sense of balance without risking a defensive attitude to anything challenging. In my experience, it is easier to lead a confident learner towards a constructively critical approach to work, than support an insecure learner to free off and have a go.

The Feel-good Factor - 3

Mistakes are cool.
They mean someone is trying.

There is no failure
Only feedback

In certain circumstances it is also appropriate to limit the learner's expectations of total success. I will often apologise for setting a particular task, *"This is really tricky and likely to cause serious problems. However it just has to be done so have a go and see what happens. You can always try again if you want to".* This is a real win-win approach.

If the task is found to be very tough there are no surprises and any problems are viewed in a proper perspective. If the task is achieved, the feeling of success is intensified because of the "this is tricky" health warning delivered at the start. Although not a technique to use too often, it is occasionally worth over emphasising the difficulties of a task in the form of an "I bet you can't..." challenge and building in success, to allow the learner the satisfaction of crowing, "You didn't think I could do that, did you? Well..." few things give me as much pleasure as seeing learners begin to believe in themselves and learning to place success and failure in their proper context.

Marking for success is a simple way to accentuate any positive aspects of work. Choosing to tick or "red pen" everything a learner does right is an interesting exercise and one which sends a very different message to one in which all errors are marked – the infamous "death by deep marking" approach. Unfortunately some teachers and many parents seem to believe that a failure to mark every error will compound the problem. This is completely to fail to understand a basic truth in marking, which is that it is pointless to mark a word like "octopus" when the learner is currently struggling with "cat"! Marking will be discussed in length later. For now it is sufficient to observe that in marking, like so many things in teaching, less is often much, much more.

3. Minimising a fear of tests

- Call them quizzes
- Give choices
- Use formative "show you know" assessments
- Throw out "I bet you can't" challenges
- Read out the questions and allow Assistants/buddies to record whispered answers
- Set achievable targets
- Teach pupils how to learn

Tests can strike fear into learners, especially those who are consistently disappointed with their achievements. In his book "Closing the Learning Gap", Mike Hughes suggests that a "quiz" always seems to be much less of a threat and there is little doubt that he is right. In fact calling it a quiz, instead of a test, can often allow the teacher to pitch an assessment at a much higher level and yield better results, simply because of the nature of the word.

Because Dyslexia is a learning difference, it follows that dyslexic learners will have different learning preferences. Therefore it makes sense to give choices within the assessment process. I find it best to invite learners to show me how much they know about a given topic and then offer a variety of "evidence" strategies linked to my awareness of their learning styles. Depending on the task possible choices could include a mind map, storyboard, flowchart, bullet points or paragraphs, with the learners choosing a style which best suits them. This flexible approach seems to empower learners to show what they know while removing artificial barriers to learning. However, the success of this approach depends on these skills being explicitly taught to mastery before being used as assessment tools.

Learners who understand how they learn seem to respond particularly well to an "I bet you can't ..." quiz situation, especially when the challenge is linked to a tangible reward – appropriate bribery can often have an important role in effective teaching! I have challenged 7 year old dyslexic learners, with very vulnerable working memories, to remember a 12 item shopping list, the challenge being, "I bet you can't get 8/12".

Providing they use their knowledge of their learning styles, these youngsters not only beat the challenge after 10 minutes learning, they can also do it again an hour later, a week later and a month later. The key to success is, of course, the combination of a realistic challenge and learners who understand how they learn best.

Marking for Success

In a paragraph:

- Tick all the words spelt correctly

- Express the correct number of spellings as a percentage of the total number of words written

In a word:

- Tick all the correct letters

- Express as a percentage of total number of words written

Feel proud!

**Evidence of Learning
"What happened during a Viking raid
– why were they so successful?"**

You can do it as:

- **Paragraphs**
- **Bullets**
- **Flow chart**
- **Story board**
- **Mind map**
- **A model**
- **"Physical theatre"**
  representation

Conventional tests usually require learners to read questions and write answers. Although the intention of the assessment may well be to test knowledge of a subject, in reality what is tested is the ability to read, formulate answers and write them down. Dyslexic learners usually know as much as their classmates but tend to have problems initially reading the questions and then processing, organising and recording an appropriate response.

The reading barrier can be easily removed by reading the questions to the class; removing the writing barrier takes a little more imagination.

One simple solution is to assess though a buddy system. This can work in several ways but tends to rely on one child whispering answers to a buddy with stronger basic skills who writes them down. After an appropriate number of questions the buddies can go on to their own assessments – paper based or whatever. This also works well with older children acting as scribes, perhaps Years 5+6 in primary schools and 6th formers at secondary.

But there is a possible danger to this approach, as this true story illustrates:

> "The Head of History in a developing comprehensive school decided to teach a group with learning difficulties in order to set a good example to his staff. After the first 6 weeks he set the unit test, a combination of multi-choice and written answers, and was devastated by the poor results. However, he soon realised that, far from testing historical knowledge and understanding, the assessment was no more than a test of reading and writing. In consequence, his dyslexic learners with currently weak basic skills were denied the opportunity to show what they knew.
>
> Another test was set, this time with a Sixth Former sitting next to each learner. The teacher read the questions, the learners whispered the answers and the Sixth Former wrote them down. When the papers were marked, an interesting pattern emerged – although the class was perceived by many teachers as being slow, difficult to teach, possibly even not worth teaching, etc, it scored more highly than a majority of pupils across the year group. They were, in fact, very good young historians with a sound grasp of the key concepts – writing it down was the only problem!"

When I tell this story, teachers often respond by pointing out that, because this is not what happens at SATs and GCSE, it is a pointless exercise. I always beg to differ because those pupils addressed future tests with a remarkable confidence and assurance. Once they began to believe in themselves they found ways to minimise their difficulties and no longer allowed tests to inhibit their thinking.

The message, I think, is that empowering children to show what they know, boosts their confidence and self-esteem to such an extent that they begin to be the best they can be, even in national examinations.

4. Minimising a fear of reading out loud

- Invite all pupils to read but build in the "right to pass"
- Promise not to ask certain pupils under any circumstances
- Allow pupils to record reading on tape/Dictaphone/speech-write
- IT programme
- Set up paired reading/group reading/choral speaking situations

Many dyslexic learners are extremely reluctant to read out loud and a common response is not to ask them to do so. While this goes some way towards addressing the issues, it is still divisive and can stigmatise learners in front of their peers. A more inclusive response is to institute "the right to pass". It works like this: all learners are invited to read whenever a task dictates. However the "right to pass" means that the invitation can be declined by anyone, preferably with a gracious "No thank you". Giving all learners the choice to read is inclusive – giving all the right to decline is supportive.

This approach may seem a trifle extreme and teachers express concerns that nobody will read. In practice this does not seem to happen, because many learners enjoy the chance to read out loud and are very good at it. Children who lack confidence in their reading seem to enjoy the right to pass – it gives them a degree of control and I have never found the situation to be abused. Some learners still feel insecure and, if this is the case, it may be better never to ask them. Experience suggests that the right to pass is so effective that, while the most reluctant readers initially clamour for the opportunity to refuse with dignity, they later surprise themselves by saying "I think I will read today". I doubt if that situation would arise had they not been able to exercise a degree of control over their activities in the classroom.

Inclusion and Empowerment
through Reading out loud.

Do we say to teachers,
    "Please don't ask ….to read
    out loud?"

Or do we say,
    "Please ask everyone to
    read out loud – but build in
    the right to pass?"

Go for:
    "The right to pass" – the
    inclusive option

There is, of course, a significant difference between reading out loud in front of peers and doing so quietly to the teacher. Regardless of age and competence, some reluctant readers prefer to come to the teacher's desk, while others are happier if the teacher comes to them. Responding to individual preferences is an important part of winning trust and developing a learner's emotional security.

For some, an ideal compromise is to read on to tape, Dictaphone, or web cam for the teacher to hear later. This sort of activity can be a useful technique to break down barriers and win trust.

Paired reading is a technique which, though often amazingly effective, is often misunderstood and thought to involve readers taking turns. It is, in fact, simultaneous reading out loud, with the stronger reader taking responsibility for cuing any tricky words. The guiding principle, during the early stages, is that the weaker reader has choice of material. This is an important point as it establishes a purpose for reading, something which is not always clear to learners – for many, reading is yet another teacher directed activity which has no relevance outside the school gates.

Choices may include horoscopes, sports/fashion/gossip pages of newspapers, magazines etc, etc. Sometimes a choice may seem inappropriate, but it is important to respect the learner's right to choose, and to make a poor choice if necessary. One of my 13-year-old pupils wanted to be a lawyer and chose a legal text from the library. We struggled through it for the session and, at the end, I asked her if she had enjoyed it. "No, not really" was the reply. "I think I'll choose something different tomorrow". Her new choice was a Mills and Boon, which one of us really enjoyed!

A little training supports the more experienced reader to be more effective. Helpful techniques involve backing off the pace to allow the weaker reader to cue the words: sometimes it is effective not to say the initial consonants, forcing the learner to cue the consonant and then being supported with the rest of the word. It may seem odd to read "the _at _at on the _at" instead of "the cat sat on the mat" but it works. However it must stop as soon as problems occur. A period of "normal" paired reading must follow to re-establish pace and confidence.

Paired reading is also an effective buddy technique for comprehensions across the curriculum. Paying attention to pairing is often helpful, especially when a sound reader, with average/low average thinking and/or reasoning skills, is paired with a weak reader with well-developed conceptual skills. This pairing often results in improved work for both partners.

Paired Reading Guidelines

1. Pair a weaker reader with a stronger reader

2. The weaker reader has choice of material – whatever s/he wants to read

3. Both students read out loud simultaneously

4. The stronger reader "carries" the flow and cues any tricky words

5. Definitely no teaching or sounding out

Encourage the stronger reader to:

- Slow down when a word is difficult

- Pick up the pace once all is well again

There can be some parental resistance to paired reading/peer tutoring due to an understandable concern that their child will, in some way, be held back by the process. In practice this does not seem to be the case. The thinking that goes into the process empowers the stronger reader to become even more effective while the weaker partner gains in fluency and comprehension – a fine example of a win-win situation.

Choral speaking is an effective variation of paired reading and one that can be very popular. Chanting information from books or board also serves to include reluctant readers in the process. Both techniques work across a variety of subjects, the only limitation being the teacher's imagination and the willingness of the group to participate. Group reading is a similar activity in which reading tasks can be shared. I prefer to stipulate how many people in each group are required to read, giving an opportunity for the less confident to pass. Inviting group members to present in unison also works, though it can be noisy as it usually seems to require a number of enthusiastic practice sessions.

Reading out loud is only a problem when it is made a problem. Unfortunately it can be teachers who create the problem in the first place and then compound it with insistence and persistence. As with most things in teaching, giving the learner a measure of control and a degree of choice goes a long way to minimising many issues.

Summary

How to create the feel-good factor through strategies which minimise:

- A fear of disapproval or lack of understanding
- A fear of failure
- A fear of reading out loud

Chapter 4

EMPOWERMENT THROUGH DIFFERENCE

The feel-good factor can support learners to feel so good about themselves that they are prepared to take risks, to have a go and believe that "mistakes are cool". However, residual anxieties may still focus on concerns about keeping up and organising their thoughts.

Particular issues may include:

- Not being able to keep up
- Information overload
- Not being able to get started with written work

1. Minimising the fear of not being able to keep up

- Differentiate by task and/or outcome as appropriate for the task

- Organise a scribe – perhaps LSA or buddy

- Set up shared writing – pupil does some of the writing

- Encourage the use of mind maps, storyboards, flow charts etc and be prepared to mark them for content and ideas

- Never, ever, under any circumstances dictate passages to be copied into exercise books in order to "cover the curriculum"

- Minimise/eliminate the requirement to copy from the board – try making a quick précis for a child to copy and then pass it on, or borrow books from pupils who have finished

Differentiation is about curriculum access and, when used in a context of learning differences, supports a learner to operate effectively within less favoured styles of information processing. Differentiation by task is often presented as the "inclusive" option.

However, this style is often perceived as stigmatizing by learners who are given a trivial task and are often given it last – it is a bit like being the last one to be chosen for a team. When busy teachers do not have the time to plan /produce three or more parallel activities within each lesson, the MSC model (see opposite) supports differentiation by task.

DIFFERENTIATION BY TASK (For empowerment and independence)

Differentiation by Task or Differentiation by MSC?

Differentiation by task is a popular "theoretical" model, especially among those in a managerial or inspectorial role. However, it can be very much less popular with practicing teachers because of the workload implications. The key to the MSC model is the preparation of a "core" worksheet that all learners must be able to access and complete, either on their own or with adult/peer support. This worksheet carries all of the key issues of the lesson in an accessible form and, if that is all that some do, then it is enough. Particular attention is paid to the reading level and learning preferences of the most vulnerable learners, while trying to offer an appropriate intellectual challenge – it is important to recognise that currently weak basic skills do not necessarily imply weak reasoning skills.

Planning the Activities

"All must"

For a majority of learners, the "all must" worksheet serves only as an introduction, giving the big picture and involving them in some review and prediction activities. However, since some pupils may need to spend all lesson on this task, it needs to carry enough "big picture" information and concepts to stand alone for some learners.

Differentiation – The MSC Model

ALL MUST: (Core element – "if this is all they do, it is ok")

- Aim task at top but access for all via oracy
- Weakest may take all lesson and finish for homework

Best past the post, move on (but not first to finish!)

MOST SHOULD: (First Extension Activity)

- Oracy activity to kick off next task
- Go for five, etc. - report to teacher before moving on
- Finish for homework

Best past the post, move on (but only if top quality!)

SOME COULD: (Second Extension Activity)

- High level extension activity - aimed at top thinkers to include some dyslexics
- Organised as for first extension.
  "High Challenge, low stress"

"Most should"

"Most should" complete the worksheet quickly and go on to the main part of the lesson. This part of the lesson is often based on standard textbook material.

"Some could"

"Some could" finish this work and go on to something even more challenging, perhaps working on material from another key stage or age range.

Best past the post"

The principle of "best past the post" is important. Learners only move on to another task when the quality of work dictates – even if they have finished quickly. Quality work is the only passport to the next activity, an important message for the more impulsive and impetuous learners.

It is also important to pay attention to the nature of the "Some Could" tasks. If they involve more of the same, it can discourage learners from finishing one written task in order to do yet another. On the other hand, if the final task involves research on the web, perhaps to develop a project or similar exciting activity, some learners may never get the opportunity to take part because they cannot finish enough tasks to qualify. It is important, therefore, to build a range of activities into all levels of the differentiation process and to use positive discrimination to ensure that all learners have equal access to a range of activities.

Differentiation by outcome

Differentiation by outcome is just that. The main theme of the lesson will be presented to all, together with group activities to take the task forward. A range of tasks follow, each task being chosen to match learners' preferences, abilities and current skill levels. Differentiation by outcome seems to get a bad press in certain educational circles and has sometimes been dismissed as "un-inclusive". When used properly I would argue that it is an important technique which is very inclusive and one that offers real opportunities to teachers and learners alike.

At its most simple, outcomes can centre on quantity of work presented; some learners will be expected to produce several paragraphs, others encouraged to write several sentences. A more creative approach is to stipulate the form in which the evidence will be presented. For example the evidence stipulated for a given task could range from paragraphs, through story boards to mind maps, either with learners having a choice of presentational style or being told what is required.

A frequent concern is that some learners will resent the apparently less challenging tasks given to their peers. This is usually less of an issue in a Dyslexia Friendly classroom where it is understood that all members have different strengths and weaknesses. When this concern becomes an issue over time it helps to insist that all learners provide evidence in a range of styles. In this way the setting of different tasks becomes an expected part of everyday lesson management.

It is also possible that some learners will feel stigmatised by being set an "easier" task. In this case it is easy to offer them something more in keeping with their self image and then, at the end, to ask them if they are happy with the outcome. If they are, then they are ready to be challenged next time. However less confident learners often appreciate being set a less rigorous task within the lesson framework because they feel included in the lesson but not over-faced. Having been set a different outcome, it is not unusual for learners to exceed expectations simply because they now approach the task with a sense of self-belief! As with so many things in teaching, it is the quality of the interaction between teacher and learner that defines the task and the success of the final outcome.

Differentiation by task and by outcome are key elements in inclusion and I believe that there is a place for both strategies, often with different learners within the same lesson.

Differentiation by Outcome
(for Inclusion and Empowerment)

- Everyone involved in planning, etc. through group work

- All hear the same message – setting the highest expectations for all

- Establish a hierarchy of finishing points

- Each finishing point chosen to provide meaningful evidence of learning

"If you are happy that this is your best work, as far as you've got is fine for me!"

Differentiation by learning styles and preferences – the "self prescribing approach"

One manifestation of Dyslexia as a learning difference is that learners often think much faster than they write. If they are to interact with lessons at an ability appropriate level it is important that they are empowered to do the thinking without being penalised for current problems with recording, etc. Carefully prepared worksheets which require a maximum of thinking, but a minimum of recording are one effective, though time-consuming, solution which is being used successfully in many schools. Alternatively, the class teacher can harness the power of peer tutoring or other buddy systems. Arranging for one learner to do some of the writing for a peer can be very effective. This is best organised so that one learner dictates to another, ensuring that the ideas and language patterns are recorded accurately. If this process leads to discussion and amendment, so much the better. A bonus is that the buddy with the stronger skills seems to gain a great deal from this process as s/he contributes to the task – this is an important point to make to parents when the matter is discussed.

Differentiation by outcome through learning styles and preferences

The "self-prescribing" approach

The key question?

"What is the best way for you to show me what you know?"

In some cases the task and subsequent mark can be a genuine collaborative effort, especially when the relative strengths and weaknesses of each individual are the basis for the pairing. For some creative tasks a divergent thinker with currently weak basic skills will be a good foil for a "straight line thinker" with strong basic skills. Equally a convergent thinker will add a sense of purpose and focus when paired with a natural "multi-tasker" when there is an optimum solution/end product.

Shared writing is a technique perhaps best used when an adult is involved and this can be especially useful when supporting a reluctant writer. Negotiation is the key here, with the adult striking a bargain with the learner regarding the amount and nature of writing each will do. Effective negotiated positions can include:

You write a line and I'll write a line
I'll do the first two lines and you do the rest
You do the first two lines – tell me the rest and I'll write it
I'll write the first paragraph and you can do the next….
I'll write the ideas on post-its/strips of paper – you organise and I'll write up or you can paste in to your book

Down with Dictation

It is difficult to find an educational justification for using dictation in the classroom if the purpose is to fill exercise books in order to "cover the curriculum". Dictation as part of a programme to develop spelling, auditory memory or with some other "therapeutic" aim is, of course, quite acceptable. Teachers report that dictation to get work into books, once only the curse of certain secondary schools, is becoming a common practice in some primary schools in response to the pressure to cover the curriculum.

The problem with dictation is that many learners can write the words automatically and have very little idea of what has been recorded. Consequently they will have to spend their time reading through in order to work out what it is that they have been "taught". Other learners find the process so stressful that they become almost paralysed and their notes are practically useless. The only person who seems to benefit is the teacher who can tick another page off the scheme of work as having been covered.

> # Down with Dictation!
>
> ## The use of dictation to:
>
> ## "cover the curriculum"
>
> ## is impossible to justify in any rational educational setting.
>
> ## Remember:
>
> ## "Education is not the filling of a pail, but the lighting of a fire."
>
> William Butler Yeats

If it is important to get a body of information into books it is far more effective to hand out photocopies to be pasted in. Learners can then be encouraged to interact with the ideas by, for example, highlighting key words/phrases and/or by summarising the ideas and presenting them in different forms. Reducing the text by a given number of words or to a number of key words is also effective. Highlighting key words and expressing them as a mind map, flow chart or storyboard requires the learner to "pole bridge" or use learning techniques which require the use of both sides of the brain, a process that is generally recognised to optimise learning. The opportunity cost of working this way is, of course, the opportunity for active, effective learning against the cost of passive copying. The printing bill can be justified as part of a best value approach and also as an observable aspect of an accessibility plan.

Copying from the board

Copying from the board, while perhaps easier to justify than dictation, can also present serious challenges to many learners. The ability to copy at a distance relies on highly developed tracking skills underpinned by stable eye movements, something which many learners do not possess. Once a learner gets past the first two or three lines, it becomes increasingly difficult for them to scan back to where they need to be. In consequence they find themselves having to go back to the top of the board and read through to where they need to be. Having transcribed the next bit they lose their place again and have to start at the top once more. Working this way requires a learner to read a board full of work many times in order to complete the copying task.

If it is essential that work is copied from the board try:

- Writing lines in different colours
- Numbering lines at each end – even if/especially if the writing is prose rather than points
- Making sure that lines 1, 3, 5 + 7 carry the key information and, having informed selected learners of this, require them to copy only those lines. This way they get the key information without having to write too much. (However if it is possible to get the key information in half the lines, it is hard to see the point of writing the rest!)
- Leave it up for a long time
- Wait until everyone has finished before rubbing it off – if this takes too long then copying from the board is not an acceptable or inclusive strategy for the class as a whole

An over-reliance on copying from the board sets many learners up to fail

Try a worksheet!

If you want to avoid certain learners having to copy from the board try:

- Encourage copying from the books of other learners
- Write a quick précis and place it in front of a pupil
- Borrow books from pupils who have finished to place in front of slower writers, while setting them another task

2. Minimising a fear of information overload

- Make instructions clear and concise
- Give one sound bite at a time
- Ask pupils to repeat/paraphrase instructions to buddy/assistant/teacher
- Thank pupils when they ask for help/clarification – every time, even if they were not listening
- Say what we want and be specific – "Write on the line" is better that "Take care with your presentation"

Dyslexic learners often experience problems with their short term and working memories, even though long term memory rarely seems to be an issue. A particular challenge is remembering what is seen and heard, in the correct order, long enough to do something with it. There also seems to be an unpredictable element at work in terms of what information becomes stored in the long term memory. A young dyslexic adult once described his memory as a net with holes of different sizes. Because of these holes he can never predict what information is caught and stored, finding himself remembering enormous and often irrelevant chunks of some topics and minute details of others. A challenge for the teacher is to direct information to the "memory net" in ways that ensure it is caught.

The way instructions are sequenced and delivered can make a major difference to the efficiency and effectiveness of the learner's short term memory. Best advice is to "think then talk" to ensure that instructions are clear, concise and unambiguous – showing learners a row of shovels and spades and asking them to take their pick may cause some initial confusion! As a rule of thumb, it is probably best to deliver instructions in one or two chunks while always remembering that, on a dyslexic day, short term memory is often down to one chunk or even less.

Take up time is also important. One opportunity cost of a differently wired brain seems to be a reduction in automaticity in certain tasks. Giving time for instructions to be processed is helpful, as is paying attention to one's body language while waiting - learners are often very quick to pick up on impatient body language and to spot inconsistencies between language and posture, especially if they have had bad experiences in the past. This inconsistency can be a major cause of stress which often reduces short term and working memory even further, perhaps to a point where learners seems to know less half way though an activity than they did when they started. This phenomenon is common in the stress of exam situations, but there can be no excuse for stress being allowed to cause this in normal lessons.

> # "My memory is like a net, with holes of different sizes
>
> # But,
>
> # I can never predict which bits I will remember"

A simple way to minimise the stress that can result from forgetting instructions is to give "praise for asking". This simple technique is effective, inclusive and in line with almost every school's mission statement because it involves treating all requests for help, guidance and clarification with respect. The most effective response to a request for repetition is a smile followed a simple "Thank you for asking. What I said was...." This is also inclusive because, as one learner asks for help, a number of others are breathing a sigh of relief because they did not know either and were reluctant to say. Once again, posture and tone are important, because an aggressive and sarcastic "Well thank you **so much** for asking," sends a very clear message that we do not ask for help in this class. Then at Parents Evening the teacher says, with a concerned expression, "S/he really must ask for help more"!

Managing selective attention

What about the learner who asks for help but who was clearly not listening when the instructions were given? Best advice is to respond as if they had been listening, thanking them for asking and giving the necessary information. While it is tempting to address the issue of not attending, it is probably better to "tactically ignore" it at this point and get the learner on task. However the learner and her/his friends know that "not listening" has been ignored, which could set a dangerous precedent for the future. My preferred strategy is to choose when to have a quiet word a little later: then I will point out that, although I was pleased that s/he asked for help, I would have preferred more attention when I was talking. Asking calmly, quietly and directly for what is required next time is an assertive and effective way of making a point, and one which spares the teacher's voice and adrenalin levels. It also makes the important point to the rest of the class that, although issues may not be dealt with directly, they will always be addressed at some point and on the teacher's terms.

The power of positive language

Another effective aspect of positive discipline is to ask for what is wanted, rather than say "Don't" or issue a general sort of "Be careful about" warning. For some reason there is a tendency to focus on the 'don't' which makes it most likely that the "don't" will be done. So saying "Take care with your spelling" is not as effective as identifying one or two key groups of words on which to focus. Saying "Make sure you use a 'y' to get the 'e' sound at the end of these words" is a helpful suggestion which, because it is phrased positively, is likely to be remembered and followed. Similarly asking a learner to aim to write at least one word per sentence on the line is more effective than saying "Don't be untidy". There are very few instructions, commands or directives that cannot be phrased as a 'do' rather than a 'don't' – it just takes practice.

Never underestimate the power of positive, affirmative language:

Saying "Do" gets it done,

Saying "Don't" doesn't!

3. Minimising a fear of **not being able to start**

- Always give paragraph starters – go "scaffolding"
- Use writing frames to get started
- Provide a mind map skeleton
- Ask assistant/buddy to write the opening sentence
- Ask the pupil to dictate opening sentence to assistant/buddy who writes it in
- Ask the pupil to make a plan and talk it though
- Present information on strips of paper to be re-ordered and then copied/stuck into book

Support through scaffolding

The term "scaffolding" is used to describe a flexible way of providing support for less-confident writers and it is a splendid technique for dyslexic learners. Scaffolding is an interesting metaphor because the support structure can gradually be dismantled until the learner is building on firm foundations, perhaps swaying slightly, but generally able to work independently.

Having struggled to "get it down on paper" for most of their school lives, many dyslexic learners go to great lengths to avoid writing – the unvoiced belief seems to be, "If I don't join the race, I can't come last!"
One way to begin to break down barriers is to create well structured error free situations, based on the principle of scaffolding, that make it impossible for the learner to fail.

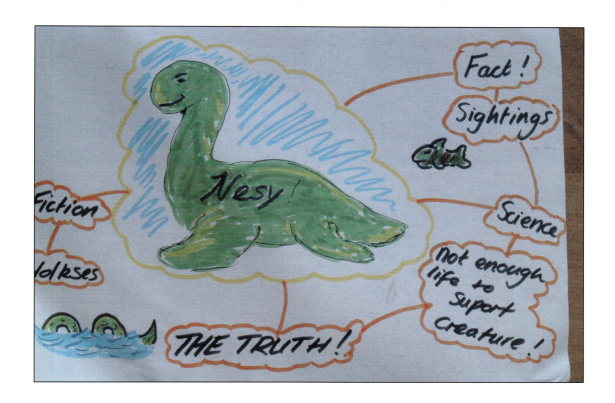

Allowing the learner to choose how to present is often very motivating –
"You mean I can do a storyboard (cartoon strip) or mind map instead of
writing? That'll do for me!"

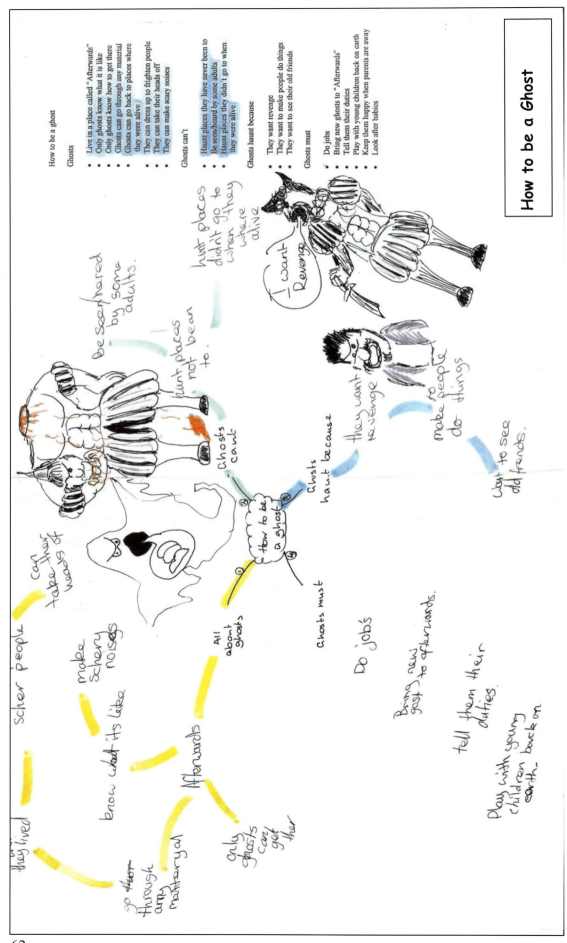

How to be a ghost

Ghosts

- Live in a place called "Afterwards"
- Only ghosts know what it is like
- Only ghosts know how to get there
- Ghosts can go through any material
- Ghosts can go back to places where they were alive
- They can dress up to frighten people
- They can take their heads off
- They can make scary noises

Ghosts can't

- Haunt places they have never been to
- Be seen/heard by some adults
- Haunt places they didn't go to when they were alive

Ghosts haunt because

- They want revenge
- They want to make people do things
- They want to see their old friends

Ghosts must

- Do jobs
- Bring new ghosts to "Afterwards"
- Tell them their duties
- Play with young children back on earth when parents are away
- Look after babies

Basic Storyboard Blank

This blank can be made using the Tables facility in Microsoft Word or by folding an A4 piece of paper the required number of times and then drawing in the lines. Try using between four and eight frames on an A4 page.

Of course doing a storyboard requires the learner to remember, organise and order information to a significant level and provides concrete evidence of thinking. With evidence like this available I often wonder why we teachers can be so insistent on sentences and paragraphs as the only acceptable forms of evidence.   Storyboards can be made more of a challenge by requiring, as appropriate, some speech bubbles or labels, in other words, to ask for some writing.

The next level of storyboard explicitly requires sentences as well as words and is set up accordingly

I usually ask for "at least" one line of writing under each picture to carry the writing forward and will sometimes require speech bubbles as well if appropriate to the task. The task can also be started by the teacher, Assistant or buddy with the learner taking responsibility for the pictures and dictating appropriate text. Once the learner is writing her/his own commentary in support of the pictures, it is a small step to ask for the sentences to be written down in prose. If the learner negotiates a deal like "I'll draw the pictures if you write what I say" then I am always happy to go with this, at least for the first few times.

When the time is right for the learner to accept responsibility for the full process, warn them at the start that this will happen, ask them how they feel about it and be prepared to back off if necessary. It is definitely not worth getting "heavy" about writing; the learner will be ready when s/he is ready and the length of time it takes to get there will depend on the damage done by thoughtless demands in the past.

It is a short step from this storyboard to asking learners to plan their thought in cartoon form and then use the plan to produce free writing in the appropriate genre.

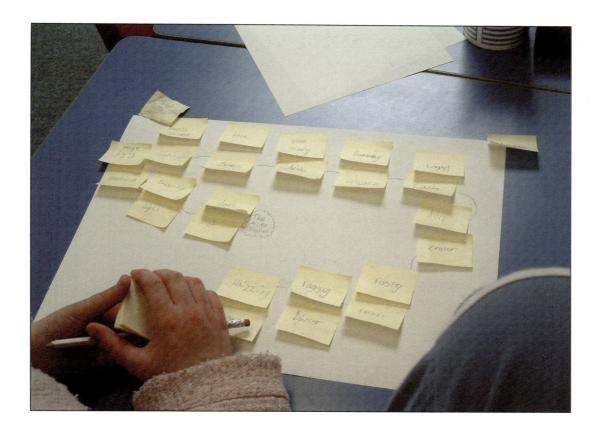

The principle of scaffolding has led learners from a "safe" representation of ideas in cartoon form, through the addition of speech bubbles and one/two liners, to a short paragraph. This technique is also very mind friendly because planning in one form and presenting in another requires the use of both sides of the brain.

The key to effective scaffolding is for the teacher to work out a possible sequence of paragraphs and the most appropriate way to start them. Although this approach may appear to limit the learner's options, in reality it frees off the thinking and allows a focus on what is to be said rather than how to start. A mind map format can also be very helpful.

The map overleaf was made using the auto shapes facility in Microsoft Word. When it is copied onto A3 paper there is plenty of room for learners to express their ideas. This particular structure works for most styles of writing, at least in the early stages of confidence building. Later the map can be presented as a skeleton, allowing learners to put their own words into the stars.

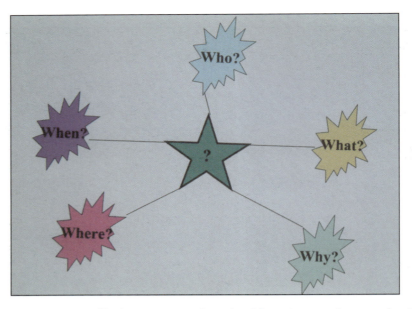

Writing frames are well-documented and effective and are a logical progression from the scaffolding techniques described above. A logical sequence of paragraph starters leads the writer towards an appropriate style of writing and effectively establishes an appropriate genre.

Starting to write can be like learning to ride a bike

Sometimes you need a helping hand to move in the right direction

Never be afraid to give paragraph starters to get the learners moving

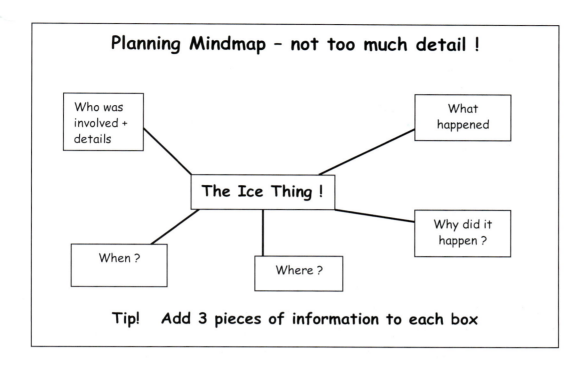

Planning Mindmap – not too much detail !

Who was involved + details

What happened

The Ice Thing !

Why did it happen ?

When ?

Where ?

Tip!   Add 3 pieces of information to each box

Hands on planning – keeping it kinaesthetic

Effective though mind maps are, they may not always help a learner who appears completely blocked. It is easy to attribute the block to a lack of ideas; however a teacher who is dyslexic pointed out to me that the problem is often due to such a wealth of ideas that the learner does not know how to choose.

Too many ideas, as well as too few, can stop you getting started as

So "I can't get started" often means "I don't know which ideas to use"

Frameworks can provide a structure which lets the ideas flow freely

One easy way to support the planning process is to work through strengths: in the case of dyslexic learners that often means building in a strong kinaesthetic and visual element. An effective way to harness the eclectic range of ideas that often typify a dyslexic learner's thinking is to use a thought shower. This technique can generate an enormous amount of information very quickly because it relies on word association and "stream of consciousness" thinking. A group of learners call out their ideas as they occur and a scribe writes the ideas down.

The key rule is that there is no evaluation, comment or discussion at this stage. This rule is important because discussion interrupts the flow of ideas. Once all the ideas have been written down, they can be discussed, modified, rejected etc. It can work like this:

- Thought shower to generate a range of ideas
- Scribe records the ideas as a list. Hot tips for easier processing include:

    1. Leave a couple of lines between each point to allow the list to be cut up for processing
    2. Write each idea on separate pieces of paper/post-its.

Although this technique is often used very effectively by teachers at the board, it is essential that learners learn how to do it for themselves as it is an important life skill. Ideas written as a list can be organised into main themes by colour coding or numbering points:

- Ideas on strips of paper can be put into appropriate heaps and then piled in possible order of use
- Each pile of strips can form one branch of a table sized mind map, allowing the "linear" information to be presented in a very

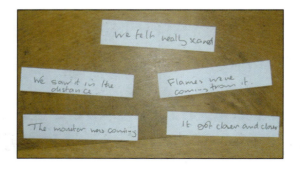

Information on strips of paper can also be used to scaffold a writing task. This time the teacher prepares information in list form and then cuts it up into strips. A set of strips is placed on each desk and the learners challenged to create the list. This approach is very effective for any linear task like, for example:

- How would you set up an experiment to separate salt and sand from water
- What happens when a volcano erupts?
- In what order did these events occur in Macbeth Act 3?
- What happened in the battle of Hastings?
- How is starch broken down as it passes through the body?
- How does a photocopier work?

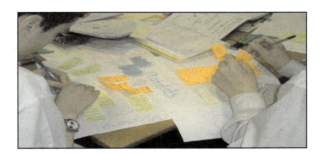

These can be turned into true multi sensory tasks. Kinaesthetic learners respond to the stimulus of handling and manipulating the strips of paper, auditory learners benefit from the discussion and decision making, while visual learners are stimulated by the pattern that is developing, especially if the strips are colour coded in the various sets. Regardless of apparent learning preference, most learners seem happy to incorporate a range of techniques in a truly multi sensory way.

Hands on

Switches

Brains on

"Keep it kinaesthetic"

When the strips have been placed in order the teacher has a number of choices regarding the final task, depending on the aim of the lesson. If the aim is to do with information selection and processing then there is no need for evidence to be presented in sentences and paragraphs. Acceptable evidence could be:

- the ordered strips stuck into the exercise books (this depends on each learner having their own strips)

- The information to be copied into the book by the pupil, a buddy or an adult

- The strips placed in the form of a mind map or flow chart and recorded on web cam or digital camera – then printed out and stuck into books (effective for group tasks)

- The strips placed in the form of a mind map or flow chart and a copy made in the exercise book

- The processed information turned into a story board, with the information on the strips either copied on to the story board or pasted on

The marking policy in a Dyslexia Friendly school will encourage teachers to offer alternative means of recording and positively encourage them to do so.

Multi-Sensory is best

The more senses involved in learning, and the more ways that information can be transformed into something else, the more permanent the learning.

There is a mistaken belief that insisting that learners always write in sentences and paragraphs gives worthwhile practice at this important skill. In reality it can prevent dyslexic learners from showing what they know and, instead of improving a basic skill, may act as a major barrier to achievement. As always, the lesson aim/objective should define the task and the evidence. Encouraging learners to "show they know" in their preferred ways, especially when they have a metacognitive understanding of their learning styles, is extremely empowering and inclusive. The Dyslexia Friendly teacher will always try to offer a choice in the way the evidence is presented because s/he recognises the importance of allowing learning preferences to define tasks.

Summary

- Differentiation by task
- Differentiation by outcome
- Differentiation by learning style and preference
- Down with dictation
- Support strategies for copying from the board
- Responding to information overload
- Power of positive language
- Managing selective attention
- Scaffolding
- Cartoons and storyboards
- Hands on planning – keeping it kinaesthetic

The Message is in the Marking

To what extent does a school's marking policy encourage or discourage learners to write at length?

"You cannot raise a man up by calling him down"

William Boetcker

Chapter 5

SPELLING WITH A SPECIFIC DIFFERENCE

Responding to spelling problems by a "Death By Phonics" approach is an automatic response in many schools, one which is actively supported by many Learning Support Teams. While few would argue the importance of phonics, it must be recognised that, like most "bottom up" methods, it can be slow, laborious and utterly boring. It also assumes that all learners prefer to learn through an auditory channel and by working from part to whole.

Unfortunately many dyslexic learners seem to be visual-kinaesthetic learners who also need to be able to see and touch what they are learning. They often seem to work best from "top down" preferring whole word to part word and resorting to chunking and syllabification as a measure of the last resort. Experienced teachers of dyslexic learners have long been aware of the danger of "putting them on a programme", in the assumption that all learn in the same way, at the same rate and with the same gaps in their knowledge and skills

However phonics as part of an eclectic response to spelling problems is likely to be much more effective, especially when good practice pervades each and every situation in which the learner is required to communicate in writing. Whole word/whole phrase reading is the holy grail – it is the way efficient readers process text. To achieve this goal, visual-kinaesthetic learners need support to develop their whole word, "big picture" skills in order to develop fluency. These skills need to be underpinned by phonic word attack strategies in order to decode unfamiliar words. Auditory/linguistic learners can "hear" the phonic elements in words and often have well-developed word attack skills. However they often find it difficult to achieve fluency because of a tendency to try to decode everything, even familiar words.

A preoccupation with mastery of phonics can also result in learners becoming "stuck" at a certain level and not being able to move on until the skills are consolidated – this is in stark contrast to some aspects of the national Literacy Strategy which puts teachers under enormous pressure to move on regardless of understanding or mastery.

The Dyslexia Friendly teacher recognises the disparity between spoken and read/written vocabulary and always looks find different ways to move learners on. For example, although c-v-c words (cat, hit etc) are key building blocks, they can be very difficult for visual learners to deal with because they all look the same – there is no shape or pattern to give clues. Perhaps surprisingly, phonically regular polysyllabic words can be easier to read and spell, especially when the words are already part of a learner's spoken vocabulary – the pattern, shape and rhythm of words like "hospital", "independent" and even "photosynthesis" can make them much more accessible than "was" or "saw".

Beware of "Death By Phonics"

Phonics may not be the best way

for visual, big picture learners!

Minimise the fear of spelling

- Never, ever, under any circumstances just say "Use a dictionary"
- Support LCWC (Look, Cover, Write, Check) with Make and Break
- Give spellings without teaching when a learner is "in the flow"
- Develop a repertoire of responses to "How do you spell….?"

  - Just give the word
  - "You try and I'll help"
  - "Can you clap it?
  - "You spell and I'll write"
  - Give the letters to "Make and Break"
  - "Are you using familiar letter combinations?"
  - Give words that rhyme

The problem with dictionaries

Saying "Use a dictionary" is probably the least helpful response a teacher can make to a spelling request, especially when a learner is in the flow of writing. The ability to find a word in a dictionary presupposes all manner of alphabetic, phonic and sequencing skills, to say nothing of having adequate working memory available as well. So, if a learner thinks that "giraffe" begins with the letter 'j', a dictionary is not going to be a great deal of help! It is also no coincidence that knowledge of the alphabet is an element of a number of Dyslexia assessment profiles since it strikes at the heart of a key area of vulnerability for many learners.

A reliance on conventional dictionaries is not very inclusive as it actively discriminates against learners with weak sound/symbol correspondence and alphabet skills. In fact conventional dictionaries condemn many pupils to a fruitless and often frustrating searching exercise which takes them right away from the task in hand and will probably discourage them from asking for help in the future.

I actually observed how the use of dictionaries can destroy a writing task when I was working with a primary school to develop inclusive writing skills. We had finished the mind maps, talked them through and the children were well into the flow of writing when the class teacher asked if she should put dictionaries on the tables. I could see no objection and the dictionaries were given out. But, as each dictionary landed on the table, the whole atmosphere altered. The climate changed from a working buzz to a pedantic, almost neurotic preoccupation with accuracy which completely killed the lesson. If I had not been there to see it I would not have believed what happened. Also the final quality of writing from this class was the poorest I had seen, both within the school and across other schools in the area where I had delivered an identical lesson.

Down with Dictionaries!

They are not a lot of help if a learner thinks "giraffe" begins with a 'j'

Also I had not become particularly aware of which children had special needs until the dictionaries arrived. Up until this point, all the children were on task and writing at length, independently and with confidence. The mention of the "D" word changed the task and completely destroyed the focus of the lesson, moving a surprising proportion of confident and independent learners into insecurity and dependence and, in a number of cases, a total "paralysis by analysis".

Just to bang the final nail into the coffin, the arrival of dictionaries did not seem to result in any great activity in terms of looking for words. Instead, the teacher was bombarded with requests for spellings. The children with effective dictionary skills could spell anyway and so did not use them, while the children with weaker skills knew that referring to a dictionary condemned them to a lengthy and often unproductive search when what they wanted to do was crack on with the writing.

This is not a case of "dictionaries are bad". However I would argue for their use in a considered and differentiated way. Choice of dictionary is also important. I have had most success with the ACE dictionary, published by LDA. It allows speedy access to words, especially when there is some doubt about the initial sounds. My ideal combination in any mainstream classroom is an ACE dictionary supported by a conventional dictionary – the ACE for quick word finding and conventional dictionaries for meaning as and when necessary.

L.C.W.C - panacea or part of the problem?

For many years "Look, Cover, Write, Check" has been used to address spelling problems. This technique is well established and familiar to many teachers who are non specialist in terms of Dyslexia. Unfortunately there is a tendency to apply it as a panacea for all spelling ills rather than address spelling issues through learning styles and preferences. This tendency is similar to the popular belief that all dyslexic learners learn best by a phonic approach, which assumes that they are all logical, step by step learners who prefer to work from part to whole through an auditory medium. As stated earlier, many dyslexic learners are eclectic learners who much prefer to work from the big picture and operate much more effectively within a kinaesthetic/visual medium.

The majority of learners in any classroom situation will have strong kinaesthetic preferences – they are the predominate group. The spread of preference within the "big three" seem to be as follows:

Kinaesthetic   37%

Auditory   34%

Visual   29%

If this is the case, any spelling technique which is not "hands on" discriminates against over 1/3 of learners in the classroom and, because of the nature of kinaesthetic people, they are not inclined to sit quietly and patiently in the face of problems/failure – they are much more inclined to fidget, become impatient and apply their creativity to finding other outlets for their talents!

Always remember the balance
of learning preferences
in every classroom

Kinaesthetic 37%

Auditory   34%

Visual   29%

To address this issue I will begin by describing the approach I have developed to respond to spelling problems. Then I will suggest some strategies for implementation in the mainstream classroom

"MAKE AND BREAK" – The MacKay Method of the whole class multi-sensory spelling

For many years I have responded to "How do you spell" requests by delving into my green bag of "Scrabble" letters and giving the learner the individual letters s/he needed. Lately, I have been using the Letter Box which is similar to the Edith Norrie Letter case and even more effective because all the letters are available for instant selection.

Wooden letters, magnetic letters and the like add a new dimension to conventional support strategies because the learner can touch as well as see during the word building process. This technique does presuppose that the learner has a degree of "sound –symbol" correspondence (knows how letter names and sounds go together) and can clap the rhythm of the word. The increased availability of small magnetic boards and letters in mainstream classrooms can add a new dimension to the technique, especially when "Make and Break" becomes house style for all learners in response to all spelling requests.

Building class responses around generic good practice is very inclusive and effective. A particular challenge will be to introduce this technique into secondary classrooms to replace the traditional "do your corrections" approach.   When the learner asks for a word s/he is given the letters in random order and asked to:

- Clap the syllables in the word several times and say it while clapping (stretching the word is also good to hear the sounds)
- Now "Make and Break":

    1. Make the word - using all the letters
    2. Break the word – into syllables
    3. Make the word – saying the syllables during the re-build and repeating as necessary
    4. Break the word – into random letters
    5. Make the word – saying letter names during the rebuild

Repeat stages 1-5 as appropriate and then follow the conventional LCWC procedure.

"Make and Break"

The multi sensory alternative to Look, Cover, Write, Check

The learner is given the letters and:

1. Makes the word

2. Breaks the word into syllables

3. Makes the word and sounds out the syllables

4. Breaks the word by jumbling up the letters

5. Makes the word – saying letter names

OPPORTUNITY/COSTS?

- The opportunity is the harnessing of multi-sensory techniques, especially kinaesthetic, to develop independent spellers who can transfer their skills across the curriculum with increasing confidence
- The cost is the time it takes to work the process through

Opportunity?

Unlike conventional approaches to spelling, "Make and Break" seems to support the transfer of spellings to different settings and subjects. For example, words learnt this way for spelling tests seem more likely to be accessed correctly during free writing situations which, as many teachers know, is not always the case for dyslexic learners. Also there does seem to be a transfer between different settings. Most teachers recognise that some learners only seem to apply spelling rules and strategies during English lessons – it is as if other lessons have a totally different orthography. However words learnt this way during, say, Geography, seem to be available for use in other subjects as well, making this technique an efficient and effective use of time.

In particular, "Make and Break" enables learners to get words into their long term memories and to access them on demand in a way that other strategies do not. This is probably because of the strong kinaesthetic and visual elements which contribute to the multi sensory whole that is necessary to accelerate the learning and recall of a word.

An analysis of the process would seem to indicate the use of the following elements:

Kinaesthetic	the tactile creation of the word and the "make and break" into syllable and letters
Visual	the shape of the word and the way the patterns develop during the making and breaking
Linguistic	the saying of syllables and letters as the word is built
Auditory	hearing the sounds/syllables as they are spoken

Mathematical/logical	the ordering of letters and sounds into a coherent whole.
Musical	the rhythm and flow of the word

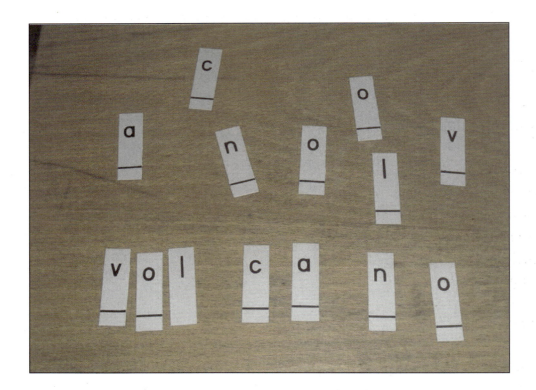

The Cost

The cost, of course, is the time it takes to work the process through compared to more familiar methods. However, since more familiar methods have been largely failing to deliver for dyslexic learners in mainstream settings, perhaps it is time to break the mould. Perhaps it is time to consider Charles Handy's definition of insanity:

> "Insanity is doing the same thing, over and over again, and expecting different results each time".

and acknowledge that, in reality, "more means different". There really is no point banging on with the same old methods just because they are familiar and/or comfortable, especially if they do not work too well!

It is interesting to discuss spelling with subject specialists in secondary schools. Most schools have a policy about literacy across the curriculum but there appears to be confusion about what should be corrected and how best to do so. Exam Boards are beginning to take a more pragmatic view of incorrect spellings which are not a "barrier to communication". While this is to be celebrated, it can risk leading to a view among teachers that, if spelling does not "count", why waste time on it?

This view can become entrenched when multi-sensory spelling techniques are suggested. A typical and understandable response is "I haven't got time for that. I can barely cover the curriculum as it is". However, because subject boards do expect their jargon words to be spelt correctly in order to achieve higher level passes, there is a clear imperative for subject teachers to use effective techniques to teach the spelling of their jargon words.

One response is to encourage colleagues to take the long term view and to consider how many times a learner will use a jargon word during her/his time in school. A word like "experiment" is required throughout a Science course and ideally needs to be spelt correctly. However, considerable time will also be spent marking the word wrong during a course of study together with well-meaning but usually ineffective ways of supporting the learning of the words – of which writing it out a number of times is probably the most ineffective. If taught in a multi-sensory way the word can be accessible for life, even for dyslexic learners. So the principle should be "right first time", investing time at the start to develop a multi-sensory "feel" for the way that complex words are constructed, especially when this feel can transfer to the accurate spelling of complex words across the curriculum.

"Make and Break" has the potential to be an effective whole school response to the correct spelling of complex, polysyllabic words. In primary settings words learnt in one year will provide a platform for other words in subsequent years, enabling each teacher to support and build on the work of colleagues. Subject specialists can invest time in their jargon words, in the certain knowledge that the generic spelling techniques they are developing will be enhanced and reinforced by colleagues across the curriculum. This, of course, is a literacy policy in action, with agreed goals being pursued by all teachers at appropriate times throughout a school year.

Spelling when "in the flow"

A "good speller" is a person who is able to access most words without having to think – automaticity seems to be the key. Dyslexic learners often see writing and spelling as two separate activities and I am regularly asked, "Do you want me to write or spell?" You can see how the learner is thinking – "If spelling is to be marked thoroughly I won't write too much to reduce the number of corrections". I tend to respond by saying that, although spelling is always important, it is more important to use the "classy words" that you use when you speak.

Therefore, regardless of the subject being taught, I will often challenge a writer to "go for it" and resist any temptation to dumb down the language in order to get the spelling right. This approach is becoming increasingly validated by exam boards in the UK through the allocation of separate marks for spelling. However, there is a very appropriate emphasis on meaning – an ambiguous spelling is more likely to lose marks than a spelling which is clearly wrong but which does convey the correct meaning.

Making multi-sensory techniques work in a busy classroom

Whenever a learner asks any question, it should initiate a "private conversation" with the teacher. Nobody else has the right to join in unless invited to do so, enabling teacher and learner to address the issues as appropriate. This is an important rule in terms of the emotional climate of the classroom; it keeps learners safe, insulates them from the consequence of sometimes naïve questions and enables them to raise issues without being put down or interrupted. Also, having finally asked for help, it is intensely frustrating when another learner blurts out the answer that had been posing a problem for so long.

Some helpful responses to "How do you spell....?"

1. Just give the word

If the learner is in the flow of writing it is often better to give the word without any "teaching". Going through a mantra of techniques at this time often results in the learner forgetting the storyline and losing the plot in

more ways than one. Teachers often find this approach a challenge at first, anticipating a deluge of spelling requests from everyone in the class. However, because "all behaviour gets you something", it may indicate some major unresolved issues in the classroom as a whole which need to be worked through in order for all to progress. For some learners, the opportunity to ask questions in order to confirm answers is part of developing emotional security and emotional intelligence.

So, while it can be frustrating to suffer "death by a 1000 obvious questions" the perceptive teacher understands that s/he is being tested for consistency of response, the logic being that if a simple question is not met with a helpful answer, what is the point of asking a difficult one?

> # Students lose more marks in exams for "playing safe" with boring but correctly spelt words than they do by "going for it," and using ability appropriate language.

2. Choosing how to give the word is important.

Depending on the learner and the situation, the following techniques offer a variety of response:

- "That is a great word – can I write it in for you" – especially helpful for complex, polysyllabic words and to support a learner who is responding to the challenge of ability appropriate language

- "I'll chunk it into syllables for you. Are you ready?" – spelling each syllable, saying letter names, offers an easy way of recording, without overloading working memory

- "The first three letters are.....etc" – works when the syllable pattern is unhelpful

- "I'll write it for you to copy" – perhaps the standard response, which can be made even more effective by challenging the learner to write the word all in one go, rather than letter by letter

Encourage them to "look to remember" and so develop visual imagery.

3. "You have a go and I'll help"

Throwing the word back in a supportive way emphasises the learner's responsibility for solving the problem. Another helpful phrase is "Which bit of the word is causing problems?" This phrase harnesses the language of possibility and encourages the learner

Encouraging learners to chunk the word develops word attack strategies in a gentle and supportive way. However this may not be appropriate for all, especially for those who currently lack confidence or who are feeling stressed by the task. In these situations it is better to give the word.

4. Can you clap it?

This is often the most effective challenge for words of two syllables or more and is particularly effective for complex jargon words. "Cool" adolescents may prefer to tap the word discretely under the table. "Stretching the word" to enhance the individual sounds also works. Try:

- giving a marble for each syllable
- dropping a marble into a tin as each syllable is heard

This method has an obvious (and delightfully noisy) self checking element. Chunking is wrong when:

- all the marbles have gone and the word has some syllables left
- the word has been completed but there are marbles left

Modelling by teacher/buddy, etc. can be particularly helpful and is a useful first step in the chunking process.

> # Helpful responses to "How do you spell....?"
>
> - ## Can I write it for you?
>
> - ## Can you clap it and say the syllables?
>
> - ## You have a go and I'll help!
>
> - ## Here are the letters – can you make and break?

5. You spell and I'll write. How does it look to you?

Offering to write while the learner dictates can reduce overload and may also serve to reinforce sound/symbol correspondence. Also the teacher's writing may be easier for the learner to read and analyse. Visual imagery seems to be a key element in developing independence as a speller. When trying to spell a difficult word most people write it in several different ways before making a decision, especially with homophones – words which sound the same but are spelt differently. The strategy works on the principle that words that look right probably are right and leads nicely into proof reading.

6. Is it using familiar letter combinations?

This follows naturally from the previous question and seeks to harness the principle of serial probability, the odds that certain letter combinations often go together. Just as reading requires the ability to crack the letter code to get at meaning, spelling is the process in reverse – building up letter combinations and encoding them to create a letter string which makes the desired sound. When marking, I will often highlight a word and ask if it says what the writer intended.

There are any number of spelling generalisations which are useful in the mainstream situation and which enables the teacher to say "If you find yourself using this combination………., you are probably wrong". Most of these generalisations are effective within the 80% rule - that is that 80% of English words follow some sort of rule. It does not help much with words like "though, through cough, plough" but it seems to take away some of the fog and mystery created by an overly phonic approach For example:

- No English word ends in 'i' except "taxi"

- The vowel combination 'ae' is almost always wrong unless you are being scientific (haemoglobin, haematite etc)

- Using 'sh' to get the sound 'shun' is almost always wrong – apart from "fashion", "cushion" and perhaps one or two more

- To get an 'ee' sound at the end of a word, it usually has to be a 'y' – "happy, silly, funny" etc. – or a double "ee" like "tree, see etc" So if you use a single 'e' to make that final sound, it is probably wrong as the 'e' is usually silent

Unhelpful responses to "How do you spell….?"

- ## Use a dictionary

- ## You can do it if you try harder

7. Give words that rhyme

Offering words that rhyme can be effective, especially when the target word does not follow an obvious rule or cannot be easily chunked. Offering "right, tight, sight" when asked for 'light' can sometimes trigger the word in the semantic store which can, in turn, support visualisation. For example, problems can occur with homophones – is it 'hear' or 'hear'? Visualisation can help here, especially if there is already a visual learning preference. So linking the word 'hear' with the picture of an ear – "Can you see 'ear' in 'hear'?" can be a useful aide memoir for some learners.

8. Look for words within words

Looking for words within words and being aware of "root word, prefix/suffix combinations" can access a number of polysyllabic words for learners with currently weak skills. In fact, providing a learner can handle phonically regular letter combinations, these pragmatic techniques can really open up spelling, especially for those who are already thinking faster than they can currently spell.

For example, the word 'department' can be accessed by building up from 'art' to 'part'. Adding the sound 'de' as a prefix takes it on a stage further leaving the addition of 'ment' to complete the word – "Well done you!"

Marking for success – a specifically different approach

Effective marking should empower the learner to do even better the next time, while taking every opportunity to develop and reinforce self esteem and confidence. Despite marking policies which emphasise the importance of target marking and perhaps directing teachers only to identify two or three errors, "death by deep marking" continues to be practiced in some schools. It is essential to understand the message for the learner which is contained in the marking.

The piece of marked work below begs two key questions:

1. In what ways does the marking encourage the writer to write at length?
2. How is the writer supported to "be better" next time?

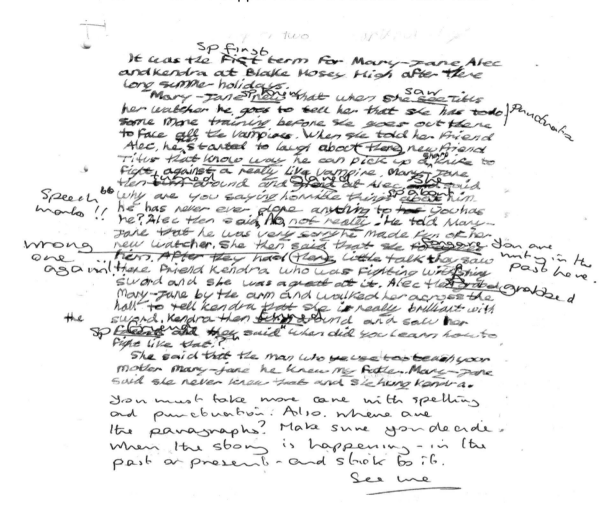

If first impressions count, the learner will be disappointed at the number of errors identified and also at the way the teacher has written all over the work. It is unlikely that the learner will be able to make much sense of the various comments because their prime function is to provide "evidence of marking" for an outside observer, parent or Inspector – rather than for the benefit of the learner! There is little chance of the next piece of work being any better, which means that the marking process was a complete waste of time!

Consider the same piece of work marked in a different way. Here the teacher demonstrates understanding of three key issues:

1. Nothing succeeds like success – so accentuate the positive

2. Learners can only handle a limited number of variables at any one time, so less marking often means more improvement – the "Less is More" principle

3. Target marking implies tactically ignoring some issues in order to focus on others. It is based on the accurate pinpointing of key issues which have been carefully selected to reflect a hierarchy of "currently achievable importance", rather than an indiscriminate and knee jerk response

(Success / Great opening sentence - wow!)

It was the Fist term for Mary-Jane, Alec and Kendra at Blake Hosey High after there long summer holidays.
Mary-Jane new that when she see Titus her watcher he goes to tell her that she has todo some more training before she goes out there to face all the vampires. When she told her friend Alec, he started to laugh about there new friend Titus that know way he can pick up a knife to fight against a really live vampire. Mary-Jane then turn around and glend at Alec, and said why are you saying horrible things about him he has never ever done anything to you has he. Alec then said no not really. He told Mary-Jane that he was very sorry he made fun of her new watcher. She then said that she forgives him. After they had there little talk they saw there friend Kendra who was fighting with shiny sword and she was a great at it. Alec then grabed Mary-Jane by the arm and walked her across the hall to tell kendra that she is really brilliant with sword. Kendra then turn around and saw her friends and they said when did you learn how to fight with that.
She said that the man who you use to teach your mother Mary-jane he knew my father. Mary-Jane said she never knew that and she hung Kendra.

(Tip - use 'there' only for where it is. Use 'their' for people.)

(Success / Some more great sentences)

(Tip: look at 'gnabed' Does it sound right?)

(Think could ya put in another paragraf?)

Great start to the story. Well done you. Please look at the tips and try to correct 1 or 2 "there / their" mistakes.
I am looking forward to the next bit!

90

> The mediocre teacher tells
>
> The good teacher explains
>
> The superior teacher demonstrates
>
> The great teacher inspires
>
> William Arthur Ward

Here, the teacher is using three key words to direct and inform the marking process:

"Success" – which is just that. It identifies aspects which are to be celebrated now and built upon in subsequent work. The teacher is saying, "I want more of this please".

"Tip" – identifies a mistake, but in a non-threatening way. The tips are points which the learner really should be sorting out independently having already shown s/he can do so in the past. The message is "I really do not want to have to keep making these points. Please sort it out".

"Think" – targets an issue for the learner to think about and make a decision.

> *This model is from "Closing the Learning Gap" by Mike Hughes*

This is marking for success while identifying a couple of "improvement issues" for next time. While there is much more that could be marked, the tips reflect current priorities that the learner can be expected to deal with independently. There is also something to think about, in terms of where a paragraph break might go. Finally the comment is positive and affirming, making it quite clear that, while the work has good elements as it stands, it will be even better if the tips are followed.

> # Bad marking wastes opportunities with feedback
>
> # Good marking "feeds forward" to make the next piece better

The important point about this style of marking is that there is very little "feed back" – all the marking "feeds forward" towards an improvement in the next piece of work. Not only does it set clear guidelines for improvements while identifying a manageable number of improvement issues, it is also much quicker and more effective.

Summary

- Make and Break – the whole class multi sensory alternative
- Spelling when "in the flow"
- Making multi sensory techniques work in a busy classroom
- Helpful responses to "How do you spell.....?
- Marking for success – a specifically different approach

Chapter 6

LEARNING STYLES AND PREFERENCES
Harnessing Learning Differences

There are at least 8 identifiable learning styles and preferences and some researchers would argue for the existence of many more. Working on the "less is more" principle, 8 learning variables are probably quite enough for the busy classroom teacher to build into an effective style of teaching and learning. It is important to think of learning styles in the plural – we all have a unique blend and it is a rare individual who is only happy in one style. Having said this, teachers need to beware of a tendency to deliver within a narrow band of styles, especially when the choice is based on one's own preference.

From personal experience I know how is easy it is to present information according to my preferences rather than how the learners need to receive it, often to the detriment of the majority of learners in a class. Although this tendency is by no means uncommon, it is easy to correct once recognised and my experience has been that most teachers react very positively when the issue is raised.

The principles are fairly straightforward: brain based learning is based on high sensory stimulation within a framework of sustained cognitive challenge. Once it is appreciated that high sensory stimulation is another phrase for multi-sensory learning, the links between "Dyslexia Friendly" and "mind friendly" become clear –more learning takes place when more senses are brought into play. Sustained cognitive challenge can be more difficult to facilitate, especially with learners who have little confidence, who suffer from low self-esteem and who currently lack strategies to tap into their emotional intelligence.

There can be a perceived conflict between developing confidence through "error free" tasks and the need for sustained challenge. This conflict is most easily resolved through self-knowledge, which is sometimes referred to as "metacognition". It enables learners to select preferred ways in which they access and present information with the twin principles of choice and empowerment combining to reduce stress.

Once learners are comfortable in a variety of styles there comes an element of "self-prescription" as appropriate methods are selected to perform the allocated tasks.

Teaching through learning styles and preferences is one way for teachers to achieve more without working any harder. Indeed it is unlikely that many teachers are able to work much harder – there is probably not very much left in the tank. If this is the case, the only way to achieve higher targets etc is to work in a smarter way – "working smart rather than hard" - and by rejecting some more traditional styles of delivery, especially those based on didactic styles, in favour of an eclectic, learner-driven approach.

All learners seem to have a unique blend of intelligences and teacher intervention can modify a pupil's intelligences and approaches to learning. Indeed there seems to be some sort of reciprocal relationship between teacher and learner as both learn to develop and apply new skills. Thinking can also be taught as a discrete skill and there are a variety of approaches available, including "Somerset Thinking Skills" (Blagg et al 1988) and an increasing number of IT based programmes.

Teaching thinking children to read and spell is usually much easier than teaching non-thinkers with good basics to think!

Thinking and intelligence both develop in stages, a fact which should have an important bearing on curriculum planning. Therefore the only "right time" for a learner to develop a given skill/concept is when s/he is ready to do so. Unfortunately this commonsense approach is difficult to sustain in the current climate. However teachers in a Dyslexia Friendly school will be encouraged to look carefully at the conceptual demands of a given programme of study and make informed decisions about the appropriateness of certain topics at certain times.

A learner who is convinced that 1 kg of lead weighs more than 1 kg of feathers is unlikely to gain much benefit from some of the more abstract and esoteric aspects of the national curriculum, at least not until s/he is able to move to a higher level of thinking. From my experience, learners seem better able to grasp abstract concepts when encouraged to function within a framework of individual styles and preferences.

> # If they don't learn the way we teach them, can we teach them the way they learn?
>
> ## Dr. Harry Chasty

Making use of Learning Styles and Preferences

It is important to state, once again, that learning styles and preferences should always be referred to in the plural. This is because most learners seem to have several preferred ways of accessing, processing and presenting information. Having said this, some learners (and some teachers) can become locked in one style, often due to feelings of stress and perhaps a lack of control – "I have my method" is a refrain sometimes heard in class and in the staffroom. Most learners, however, respond to an eclectic mix of styles and it is essential that a range of competencies are developed as part of any curriculum access strategy. As a general rule of thumb, the use of more learning styles tends to equate with more learning.

The 8 Learning Styles – keeping it simple!

1. Kinaesthetic – "body smart"

As many as 37% of most classes in school are likely to be kinaesthetic learners, forming the largest group across the range of preferences. Although the predominant group, these learners are arguably the least well equipped to operate outside of their strongest preference for long periods of time. They need to get their hands on what they are learning and are particularly effective when processing information on flash cards, post-it notes and strips of paper. Kinaesthetic learners tend to remember what they do. This group of learners often seem to prefer to organise their information in linear, logical ways, a preference particularly suited to paper based materials. Movement is very important for these learners: "institutionalised fidgeting" (giving opportunities to fiddle quietly and unobtrusively) and aspects of Brain Gym can often mediate a task which is currently being presented in a non-kinaesthetic way.

> # Thinking and intelligence develop in stages. The only "right time" for learners to develop a given skill or concept is when they do

Development Strategies

Developing strategies for movement offers opportunities for a change of state, which can be a key part of the learning process. Most adults recognise the importance of physical activity when engaged in learning and it is important to instil the habit in young learners. Telling a learner to get up and walk around while processing information could seem like a recipe for disaster, yet it can often be an effective strategy; Brain Gym for all is also likely to be effective, especially during preparation for and just before/just after an assessment.

2.   Auditory/Linguistic - "word smart"

Auditory/linguistic learners are traditional learners, forming approx. 34% of a given class, and they are well-suited to a didactic style of teaching. They tend to remember what they hear and learn particularly well when they are required to explain ideas to others. Reading information out loud and explaining to others form the bedrock of this learning style, as does a preference for information to be presented in an eclectic way. They are also fortunate in that their preferences seem to be actively promoted by the inspection process and by national exams throughout the Key Stages and at GCSEs. Furthermore there is often a perception among teachers that the auditory style is the easiest in which to deliver. It certainly seems to be a preferred choice in response to pressure to "cover the curriculum".

Development Strategies

This important preference needs to be developed to a level of competence and familiarity in all learners. Explaining processes and ideas to others are helpful activities, as are peer tutoring opportunities. "Tell your partner what you have to do/how you did that…" are valuable tasks, as are memory games and telling stories. Encouraging learners to develop their own mnemonics is also valuable. Formal opportunities to present to the class may not always be appreciated but can, with all due help and support, begin to develop auditory/linguistic skills in many vulnerable learners. Barrier games also help to develop speaking and listening and the communication of step by step processing.

> # Alice was an auditory learner, when she was in Wonderland
>
> # She said "I don't know what I think until I hear myself say it"

3. Visual/Perceptual - "picture smart"

Visual/perceptual learners are reported to form around 29% of the learning population and need to draw diagrams, charts, cartoons etc in order to "lock" their learning. Faced with "death by dictation" visual learners much prefer to have the transcript in front of them and to highlight information in different colours to represent main ideas, themes etc. This is also an excellent activity to introduce mind mapping.

In fact nearly all learners seem to process information effectively in this way, even the colour blind, who come up with combinations of colour/shading to suit their perceptual needs. Colour association can also play an important part in the recall of information while information processing techniques based on concept mapping can form an important part of a revision strategy. Most visual learners report the ability to think in pictures and some actually seem to think in video!

Development Strategies

Much of the brain is dedicated to visual processing so supporting the ability to visualise and use imagery is a key element in learning and recall. Visual skills can be developed by actively teaching information processing based on highlighting, colour coding and visualisation. Concept mapping is another important technique – in fact it is arguably the most effective way in to information processing for all learners, regardless of learning preferences. This assertion will be developed later.

4. Logical/Mathematical – "number smart"

Mathematical/logical learners are step by step thinkers who prefer to work within a logical structure. Often precise, abstract thinkers, they enjoy linear processing and problem solving which is reflected in their preference for orderly note taking. Processing information with flow charts is often a preference, once the skill has been developed.

Development Strategies

This preference is an important one to develop with all learners as it compliments most of the other styles. It can be used to develop prediction exercises across the curriculum by asking, "What would happen next if/when...". This supports learners to develop problem solving skills and to begin to process information in a logical manner. Practical experimentation is also helpful, especially when learners are required to express their findings in a step by step way. Information on strips of paper. flash cards and post-it notes supports the development of mathematical/logical techniques.

> Presenting information on strips of paper or post-it notes opens up multi-sensory opportunities across the range of learning preferences

5. Musical – "rhyme and rhythm smart"

Musical learners are sensitive to rhythm and rhyme and are particularly influenced by the emotional content of their learning. Linking information to emotions is a powerful technique and one which seems to benefit most learners. The power of musical learning can be witnessed by the ability of children to pick up lyrics as soon as a new song has been released by a favourite performer. It is also no coincidence that much early language work is done with song and rhyme, something which is also a key part of most effective work in MFL and EAL. Most of us learn tables and other chunks of sequential information through rhythm, perhaps chanting and clapping to develop a rap.

Development Strategies

Musical learning can be supported by requiring learners to look for rhythm and rhyme in words, phrases and general learning and to present information in the form of a rap or even a tune. The process of selecting background music to go with the beating of the heart may help to remember the flow of blood through the chambers and creating a mnemonic or a rap can be effective when learning a variety of information in a range of subjects. As with all styles of learning it takes practice, persistence and the opportunity to make mistakes before arriving at optimum solutions.

6. Interpersonal/Social – "people smart"

Interpersonal/social learners enjoy working with others and operate particularly effectively in group situations. Often good mediators, they can be skilful negotiators and seem to enjoy the opportunity to present their ideas to a wider audience. Cooperative learning situations can be a particular strength, though staying on task may be less so!

Development Strategies

With almost all job adverts requiring "good team players" it is essential that all learners develop competent people skills. Yet this can be a challenge for many, especially those who prefer to think in a linear fashion and who become frustrated by any perceived lack of direction in the group setting. Cooperative learning and peer tutoring activities strengthen interpersonal skills, as do pair/share scenarios. Supporting learners to become effective members of a group is important as is encouraging the group members to develop support skills of their own. Assessing a group on the performance of their most reluctant participant is a risky business but it can benefit all concerned, given appropriate ethos, culture and support mechanisms.

7. Intrapersonal/Intuitive – "self smart"

Interpersonal/intuitive learners seem to have a clear idea of their strengths and abilities and are motivated by an inner drive. Often private people, they are sensitive to their own values and prefer to be allowed to work in their own ways. Although not always the most flexible or eclectic of learners, their "self smart" skills can enable them to work independently and with great persistence and motivation. However they can feel vulnerable or even disenfranchised in group situations and may need to be "built up" and supported in order to operate effectively in linguistic and/or intrapersonal settings.

Intrapersonal learners
     – like do it on their own

Best advice – don't be too quick
     to go into group work

Allow time for introspective
reflection and consolidation of
ideas before sharing

Development Strategies

The ability to take control of one's learning is an important strength and one which has clear benefits across the spectrum of learning preferences. Giving time for inner reflection is helpful, especially just before moving into groups. I am probably too quick to move straight into group work without giving time for reflection and focus. Requiring learners to come to group work with their own ideas/strategies formed during a period of introspection and reflection seems to focus the group activity and empower all to make ability appropriate contributions.

8. Emotional – "I'm smart"

Emotional learners feel safe and secure and have a clear idea of their balance of strengths and weaknesses. The possession of an inner belief, based on success and respect, enables many learners to operate comfortably outside of their natural comfort zones because of an inner strength developed through prior success and empowerment. Positive self-esteem seems to be a common attribute, as is the ability to learn from failure without becoming unduly discouraged. When faced with difficulties, emotional learners seem able to recall past successes and derive strength and direction from these memories. This perhaps explains why all learners need to begin work in their comfort zones before being challenged to move out.

Development Strategies

Every opportunity must be taken to strengthen emotional literacy at all levels of ability and need as it is arguably the most important of the learning styles and preferences. The other styles rely upon emotionally literate learners to select the appropriate methods and to work with passion and enthusiasm. Developing a passion for learning usually begins from a platform of emotional security and success, working from within comfort zones and, if necessary, within an "error free" learning environment. Language is also important, especially the language of success (both spoken language and body language) which communicates faith in the learner, acceptance of outcomes and optimism for the learner's future. "Your best is good enough for me. Every time you are proud of your work it will take you forward".

Summary

- **The 8 styles of learning**
- **Issues for learning and development strategies for each preference**

Chapter 7

LEARNING STYLES AND COMFORT ZONES: working from inside out

Putting it all together – VAK or KAV?

The three main preferences are usually represented by the initials VAK, representing visual, auditory and kinaesthetic styles. I feel that it is more accurate to think in terms of KAV, because kinaesthetic learners tend to form the majority in most classes, with the division between styles being about 37% kinaesthetic, 34% auditory and 29% visual as stated earlier. This should be viewed with a degree of caution and the preferences are perhaps no more than simple expressions of "comfort zones".

Furthermore few learners seem to have problems moving between a range of styles, provided that opportunities are given to start within a zone of comfort and then move on. Difficulties seem to start when learners are always required to work in areas of perceived weakness; here a lack of competence or familiarity may inhibit them from relaxing into a comfortable way of working. This may be observed in the classic SEN approach of giving learners more of what they cannot do in order to get better at it.

Perhaps the key principle of working with learning styles and preferences is through direct teaching, taking time to develop skills and techniques across the range of preferences. This approach will empower learners to move from areas of strength to areas of weakness with confidence and certainty.

Touching and Looking - The Case for being more multi-sensory

Kinaesthetic Learners

Anecdotal evidence and classroom observation suggest very clearly that the majority of learners perceived as having special educational needs at KS 2, 3 and 4 are actually kinaesthetic learners.

This begs an interesting question: are kinaesthetic learners somehow less intelligent than others, or are they are not being taught the way they learn?

My experience suggests that the willingness and ability of teachers to meet the needs of kinaesthetic learners seems to diminish as pupils get older. If this is the case, the well publicised dips in performance between key stages may be more of a miss-match between teaching and learning styles rather than any lack of actual skills. Unfortunately kinaesthetic learners become restless, fidgeting and tapping and seeming to simmer with pent up energy when their kinaesthetic needs are not met. This may be a particular problem with boys who, although making up some 50% of any school population, are over-represented in SEN groups, "bottom sets" and in exclusion figures etc. Many dyslexic learners appreciate the opportunity to work kinaesthetically as the skills required match many of their learning preferences.

The Challenge?

Developing skills and techniques across the range of preferences, empowering learners to move from areas of strength to areas of weakness with confidence and certainty.

Visual Learners

Visual learners are a significant minority who are "over represented" among many learners with diverse needs and, alongside those with kinaesthetic preferences, form a solid 66% of pupils who are non – traditional learners.

Their ability to "see what we mean" is a powerful tool for learning and one which forms a splendid platform from which to launch other ways of processing information. However they too are vulnerable in a didactic teaching environment as they quickly seem to switch off when visual abilities are not brought into play. However visual learners will often produce the most creative doodles by way of compensation.

A word to the wise

We marginalise kinaesthetic and visual learners at our peril because this majority group's need for a tactile and visual education remains undiminished and often unfulfilled right through school. Yet the problem can also become an opportunity.

There is a significant improvement in results awaiting any school which chooses to operate in a more visual- kinaesthetic way:
- The potential to meet more needs in mainstream settings
- Reducing the IEP burden
- Providing higher quality support for the weakest pupils!
- Clear evidence of the Inclusion Policy being translated into practice

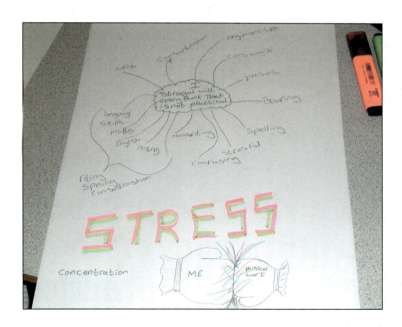

This mind map was drawn by a visual-kinaesthetic learner during a revision skills workshop. He drew it to express his frustration at the way he was expected to work in school. The task was to use the technique as a revision tool but he needed to get something off his chest first. I was able to compliment him on his use of the technique and I encouraged him to transfer this skill to other areas of learning. However he found it difficult to accept positive comments since my remarks were at odds with his view of himself as a learner and it was also clear that school had been a profoundly unsatisfactory experience for many years. It would have been interesting to talk to his parents about his early years in school. I would not have been surprised to find that, at KS 1, he was probably making ability appropriate progress in a colourful "touchy/feely" learning environment.

The Opportunities?

- The potential to meet more needs in mainstream settings

- Reducing the IEP burden

- Providing higher quality support for the weakest pupils!

- Clear evidence of the Inclusion Policy being translated into practice

It probably started to go wrong for him at about age 8-9 when visual-kinaesthetic teaching and learning styles became marginalised by more traditional methods in order to ensure full coverage of the curriculum by the end of the Key Stage. This was the point at which his learning difference became a learning difficulty. Transfer to secondary education is likely to have compounded difficulties, forcing him to work outside of his comfort zones for almost his entire timetable, the only light relief coming from subjects like PE, Drama and Technology. I got the impression he was resigned to "serving his time" with no prospect of an early release for good behaviour – so good behaviour may not always be the order of the day! However he stayed focussed for 3 hours with an unfamiliar teacher and did everything asked of him with good grace and application, presumably because he was encouraged to work from inside to out, working from his preferred visual-kinaesthetic style to whatever other styles the task dictated. He has my respect.

Linking the preferences– a whole class strategy

One of the apparent paradoxes of basing teaching on learning styles and preferences is that, even within the main three preferences (VAK/KAV) whichever style the teacher is using, 60+% of the class do not like it! The short answer is to use all three at every conceivable opportunity.

Consider the following task:

> As part of a Geography lesson the learner is asked to explain how a volcano erupts. This sort of tasks places demands on working memory (auditory and visual sequential memories) and information processing, precisely the areas in which dyslexic learners are vulnerable. Yet during the oral part of the lessons it may be quite clear that the dyslexic learners have an ability appropriate understanding of what happens and, given an appropriate learning medium, are perfectly capable of showing what they know. However being non-traditional learners along with a majority of the class, they are unlikely to be the best they can be during a traditional pen and paper exercise. The challenge facing the teacher is how to provide evidence of learning in a way which will support all learners.

One simple response is to base most information processing around kinaesthetic preferences because the nature of activities invariably engages the learner in a wide variety of tasks.

It can work like this:

- Prepare a list of all relevant (and some not so relevant) information
- Cut into strips,
- Place in envelopes
- Share envelopes between tables or pairs or whatever.

The initial task is to sort the information in terms of process, order and relevance and consideration may also be given to "piles for paragraphs" at this time. "Piles for paragraphs" simply means a loose clustering of information according to some vague initial criteria – perhaps things happening "above/below ground" as a starting point.

Use learning styles and preferences to:

- Provide evidence of learning in a way which will support all learners

- Empower them to "show what they know"

- Differentiate by outcome

A casual audit of learning styles may reveal the potential for the following preferences to be harnessed by all group members at any given time:

Kinaesthetic	– physically sorting the information into sequence and/or piles
Auditory/ Linguistic	– discussing/justifying organisation and sequence of information
Visual	- colour coding the information – e.g. brown for below ground, red for above and/or illustrating certain points on the strips with quick sketches
Mathematical/ Logical	- achieving an appropriate order of events to fulfil the task
Interpersonal	- working on delegated tasks within the group and reporting back
Intrapersonal	- making individual decisions, perhaps based on research and then reporting back
Musical	- creating the "volcano rap" as an aide memoir

Similar opportunities derive from information generated by the group during a thought shower. Most teachers use this technique as a class activity to generate information, with the teacher recording on the board. It is even more effective as a small group activity in which the group members accept responsibility for the generation and recording of information to resolve a given issue.

It can work like this:

- Each group nominates a scribe to record ideas
- The teacher sets a problem to be addressed by each small group
- Group members whisper their ideas to the scribe, who writes them down as fast as s/he can

Possible problems to be solved:

- You are astronauts about to land on an unknown planet. What can you see as you come in to land?
- How does Charles Dickens build up and maintain suspense in "The Signalman"?
- What are the implications of maintaining our reliance on fossil fuels?

- How many uses can you think of for one house brick?
- What happens to a Big Mac as it passes through the digestive system?

The task is to generate as much information as possible within a short period of time and then to process it according to set criteria. For example the teacher may ask for the three or five most important, unusual, or scary issues found by the group. Up to this point dyslexic learners are fully included in the lesson because they can express their specific learning differences as preferences in the way the information is processed. For example the list could be colour coded according to agreed criteria or it could be cut into strips and processed kinaesthetically perhaps as a list, flow chart or mind map. Also ideas could have been written directly on to strips of paper/post-its by the scribe as the information was generated. The continued inclusion of dyslexic learners depends on where the task goes next and how the next stage is launched by the teacher.

Brainstorms or Thought Showers support learners to generate information in an inclusive and enjoyable way

Key principle?

No discussion, "shout out and write down"

Dyslexia Friendly Evidence of Learning

If the lesson aim is to produce and process information on a given topic or aspect, the evidence of learning is on the table in the form of a colour coded and/or numbered list or perhaps a flow chart or mind map using strips of paper. The evidence can be recorded on digital camera or web cam etc and the lesson can move on. However it is likely that the teacher will require evidence in exercise books in order to generate individual marks and it at this point that the "dyslexia friendliness" of the lesson will stand or fall.

The least Dyslexia Friendly option is to ask for some form of write up, in sentences and paragraphs. Even though the aim of the lesson makes no mention of the need for "flowing prose" it may be difficult for teachers to break free of this traditional response to producing evidence of learning.

Yet individual evidence of learning within the tasks above could also embrace:

- mind maps
- storyboards
- flow charts
- bullet points
- scribed work
- web cam/video oral presentation

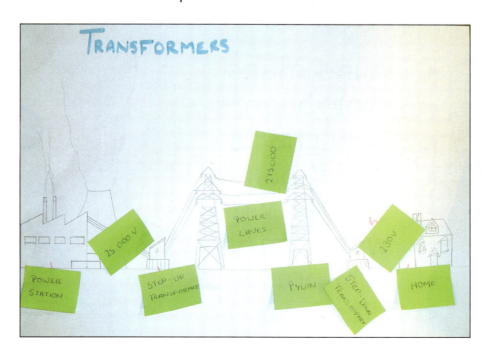

I would argue very strongly that all of these are acceptable evidence of the effective generation, selection and processing of information. Furthermore, they are within the reach of dyslexic learners whose specific learning differences empower them to operate effectively in some or all of the tasks above.

While writing in paragraphs may be a step too far for some learners, insisting that the ideas can only be presented as a story board will intimidate and even alienate others. The Dyslexia Friendly, mind friendly and inclusion friendly approach is to offer the opportunity to produce evidence in a variety of forms, allowing learners to select the one best suited to their pattern of preferences and the demands of the task. It could be that paragraphs are the most effective way to present the information and a dyslexic learner may choose to work in a less comfortable zone in order to meet certain criteria. However the key word is "choose." Working outside of comfort zones is always less uncomfortable when it is the learner's choice to do so.

Sometimes it is impossible or inappropriate to offer choice, perhaps when preparing model exam answers etc. The priority here is to ensure that learners have had the opportunity to process and handle information within their comfort zones before being expected to present in paragraphs.

Dyslexia Friendly Evidence of Learning:

- mind maps
- storyboards
- flow charts
- bullet points
- scribed work
- web cam/video
- oral presentation
- diagrams

Identifying Learning Preferences

There are a number of questionnaires available in books and on the web which can give an indication of learning styles and preferences, e.g. Advanced Study Skills by Ostler & Ward. At a mainstream classroom level, it should be remembered that there is little mystique and definitely no rocket science to working out how learners prefer to access and process information. Below are three of tricks of the trade:

1. **Visual learners** – tend to look up when memorising or recalling from memory. Looking up helps to access the visual centres of the brain and explains why flashcards should be held high and key words mounted near the ceiling. Unfortunately this need to look up while processing can lead to them being criticised for not paying attention – "The information is on the board, not the ceiling!" If you show a picture or diagram and then ask for it to be drawn from memory, visual learners will often look back at the empty board or screen, a sure sign that they are visualising the object.

2. **Auditory learners** – tend to look down and often seem to listen with their "favourite" ear, sometimes twisting their body to do so. They too may be criticised for their need to reflect their processing preference with their body language. "Face the front and look up – the answer is not on the floor!" They may express agreement with phrases such as "I hear what you are saying" and may even prefer to close their eyes to concentrate on the auditory message.

3. **Kinaesthetic learners** – tend to fidget, wriggle and communicate through gesture. They have a low threshold of boredom and will be vulnerable in didactic situations. "If it's touchable, it's teachable" for kinaesthetic learners, and fidgeting seems to aid concentration. As with the other two styles, this need to be active can be misinterpreted as wilful bad behaviour rather than as an expression of a learning preference. Institutionalized fidgeting ("blu-tac", worry beads, paper clips to bend etc) are useful management strategies. Try supplying "blu-tac" or plasticene to squeeze and squash, paper clips and even worry beads.

4. Change the task – until classroom management issues calm down. As a very general rule of thumb I find that problems with a class often result from a miss-match between the task set and the learning preferences of the group. Changing the task, either to allow more choice or to permit the use of a range of learning styles, is usually the key to success.

> # The key word is "choice"
>
> # Working outside of comfort zones is always less uncomfortable when it is the learner's choice to do so

Identifying and using the "Comfort Zones"

Comfort zones are the learning styles and preferences that suit a given learner - s/he is "comfortable" working in these ways. Given a choice, many dyslexic learners are most comfortable when working in a visual and kinaesthetic way and seem to produce ability appropriate evidence of learning quickly and efficiently through mind maps, story boards and similar strategies. However, while providing evidence in the form of sentences and paragraphs can be difficult and very uncomfortable, it is essential for exam success.

The challenge for the Dyslexia Friendly teacher is to find ways of moving learners from the zone of comfort, through the zone of challenge until they become independent learners who bring a variety of strategies to their zone of confidence. It works like this:

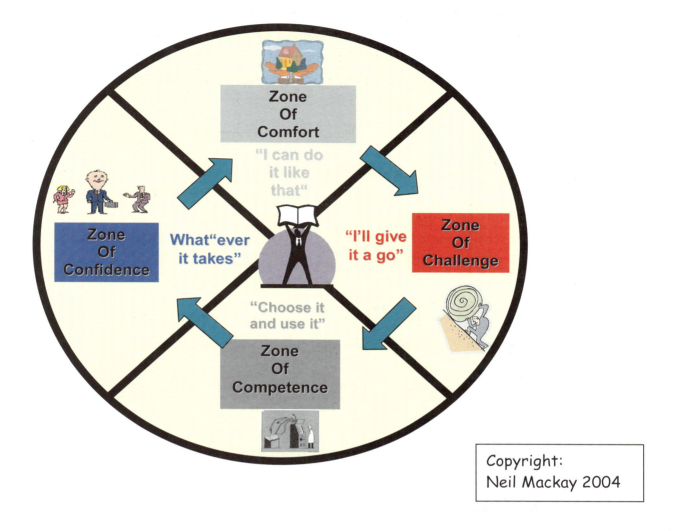

1. The Zone of Comfort – "I like to do it that way"

The comfort zone is the place where success is almost guaranteed because the learner is working in preferred ways, using strategies that s/he knows will work. It is a rewarding place to be because the tasks are designed to be delivered in an error free environment. The choice of evidence of learning in the comfort zone depends entirely on an individual's learning styles and preferences and the teacher may choose to differentiate by outcome. An eclectic range of evidence from the group could include:

- Visual learners – story board, mind map or cartoon (visual metaphors)
- Kinaesthetic learners – processing information on strips of paper or through drama/role play, making a model

- Auditory/Linguistic learners - amanuensis/ tapes/ web cam/video of discussions/role play explanations to peers, mnemonics
- Mathematical logical learners – bullet points, flow charts, information on strips of paper
- Musical learners – a rap, "rhythm and rhyme"

2. The Zone of Challenge – "I'll give it a go"

Consistent and regular success in the comfort zone empowers learners to move to the zone of challenge. Pleasant though it is to be able to choose how to present evidence, it does not reflect the reality of examinations etc. Also preferred styles may not necessarily be the most efficient or effective for a given task.

For example, although a mind map gives a very powerful "big picture" it may do so at the expense of detail: in some circumstances bullet points, a flow chart or another linear technique may be better suited to the planning and delivery of a given task.

The trick is to move to challenge from a platform of comfort and success through a series of "I bet you can't" challenges. For example:-

"That is a great mind map. I bet you can't:

- Make it a set of bullets?
- Turn it into a story board?
- Present the information as a flow chart?"

Transforming information from one form to another is a powerful way to cement learning, especially when to do so is slightly "uncomfortable".

However the mental engagement necessary to process the information into another form is essential to the future development of an eclectic and metacognitive learner. In a primary setting the class/subject teacher needs to accept responsibility for explicitly teaching each technique to mastery – in the secondary environment, different subjects promote mastery through different techniques.

What is essential is that learners have had the opportunity to practice different information processing techniques on a number of separate occasions before they are required to move out of their comfort zones and into the Zone of Challenge.

3. The Zone of Competence "Choose it and use it"

Learners working in the Zone of Confidence are given a number of appropriate strategies for information processing and are required to make a choice based on the demands of the task and the nature of evidence required. Having been empowered to develop competence over an eclectic range of strategies the learners may be able to move more readily out of their comfort zones and choose from a range of acceptable evidence producing strategies. Although perhaps less comfortable in the chosen style, the learners have weighed the opportunity costs and elected to work in a certain way in order to harness perceived benefits. Thus a learner with a mathematical/logical preference, who is most comfortable when working in a linear style, may perceive the benefit of using a mind map in order to generate the big picture. Although not within the natural zone of comfort for this learner, the mind mapping process will help to ensure that all the main issues are identified and addressed before chunking down to the detail.

The teacher has a particular responsibility to encourage and support learners to experiment with appropriate styles of information processing - and then to demand competence to be developed and demonstrated across a range of techniques.

4. The Zone of Confidence "Whatever it takes"

While the zone of confidence may include working within preferred learning styles, learners in this zone are eclectic and have a sound appreciation of metacognition. Because they understand the importance of transforming text into different forms and are experienced in the use of a variety of planning and recording techniques, they can pull down the most effective technique to get the job done. Often the method chosen will be slightly uncomfortable, but the confident learner balances the pain against the gain, secure in the knowledge that the transformation process is consolidating and extending learning.

Dyslexic learners as young as age 7 have demonstrated the ability and willingness to work through the zones and to deliberately become "uncomfortable" in order to achieve a specific result.

"Taught is not learnt"

Teaching for mastery requires repetition, practice and a significant investment of time

BUT

the results will justify the investment!

Summary

- The 8 learning styles or preferences
- Issues for learning and strategies for development
- The balance of preferences within a class
- Touching and looking – the case for being more kinaesthetic
- Linking the preferences – a whole class strategy
- Working through the zones
- Dyslexia Friendly evidence of learning
- Identifying learning styles and preferences

Chapter 8

DYSLEXIA FRIENDLY
MEANS INCLUSION FRIENDLY
Meeting diverse needs in mainstream settings

There is a perception among many teachers that a move towards inclusion places increasing burdens on the school's ability to meet special needs. What is definitely true is that we have always had pupils with a wide range of needs, especially Attention Deficit (Hyperactivity) Disorder (AD(H)D, Asperger's Syndrome and Dyspraxia/DCD as well as those who are dyslexic. Learners who are more able and talented as well those with moderate learning difficulties or emotional/behavioural issues also have learning differences which quickly become difficulties when needs are not met.

Inclusion

"There is nothing so unfair as the equal treatment of unequal children"

Thomas Jefferson

The inclusion debate offers the opportunity to review the way we identify and respond to those with diverse learning needs – that is to say, most, if not all learners in a school. It is helpful to view these needs in terms of specific learning differences and, as with Dyslexia, to base classroom responses on the continuum of learning styles and preferences. While this is not to deny the importance of discrete small group/1:1 support as needs dictate, viewing needs as learning differences is important because it directs and informs the work of the class/subject teacher for the 90+% of the time learners are in mainstream settings with non-specialist teachers (non-specialist in terms of SEN qualifications).

However, to return to the theme developed earlier, most teachers are already working as hard as they possibly can and have little time and energy left to develop their expertise in ever growing areas of pupil need. Fortunately it is possible to identify generic elements which will transfer across teaching style, lesson delivery and classroom management, rather than asking teachers to work even harder to become experts in a wide variety of learning needs. Before identifying the generic elements it will be helpful to examine discrete issues relating to each need and to identify some management strategies.

1. Attention Deficit (Hyperactivity) Disorder

The issues

Learners with AD(H)D are often warm and empathic. Great energy and enthusiasm is also typical and they are often charismatic and very effective with people. It is likely that many top sales and advertising executives have the condition to some degree because it confers the ability to focus on all the cues and to know exactly when to close the deal. In the classroom, however, this learning difference is marked, among other things, by a reduced ability to listen to instructions and to turn them into positive action.

Unfortunately this tendency is shared by quite a considerable number of learners, some of whom quite simply choose not to pay attention at a given time. The separating factor is distinguishing "won't" from "can't" – if a media star visits the school, learners with AD(H)D may continue to experience attention problems, while the "wannabes" will hang on every word, their lack of attention at other times is the result of choice and conscious decision.

The condition is often marked by impulsivity, especially with regard to shouting out and "saying then thinking". Matching activity levels to situation can be a challenge, for example talking too loudly before the start of an assembly and problems with recognising or anticipating the possible consequences of their actions can be a key issue for the management of behaviour.

To compound the issue, it has been reported that some learners actively reject any management strategies because their hyperactivity makes them feel "alive" and also makes them peer group leaders. However other learners are acutely aware of their vulnerability in certain situations and are prone to low self-esteem. Also they can become provocative victims as classmates become exasperated with interruptions and interference.

Classroom Management

The top tip is to accept the behaviour as part of the learner – although management, diet etc will help, the impulsive behaviour will always be just under the surface. However it is only a problem if made to be one. I observed a lesson where a boy with AD(H)D spent the maths lesson with his head on the table shouting out the answers. His answers were nearly always right and the teacher managed him superbly with a combination of "tactically ignoring" and giving praise for particularly good answers.

Choice of language is important, especially setting tasks and class rules in "positive language". Telling learners what to do rather than what not to do is a key skill in managing behaviour and one which transfers to all classroom management issues. So asking a learner to "read the next question/sentence" will be more effective than a general request to pay attention or stop looking around, just as "Put your pen down please" is likely to be more effective that "Stop fidgeting". It is also important to make sure the "active" part of the instruction is in the first sound bite. Saying "I'm sick of telling you and if I have to tell you again there will be trouble – stop fidgeting" easily overloads the learner who may find it impossible to separate the instruction from the emotion. A simple "Do" rather than a "Don't" is usually best.

Re-directing and getting the learner back on task without becoming locked into a "nag cycle" is another effective technique. The science of Transactional Analysis suggests "warm adult" to be the most effective communication style, the least effective being "corrective parent" – sounding like an angry or frustrated parent/carer is to be avoided at all costs, regardless of any perceived provocation! Phrases like "That is a good sentence. Please read it to me. Now carry on writing and don't stop until you have finished the paragraph" carry all sorts of messages for the learner but, because they are expressed in positive rather than negative language, the chances of success are much higher.

ADHD as a learning difference

Learners with this condition can usually think as well as other children at the same level of ability – the challenge for the teacher lies in empowering the production of ability appropriate evidence. Learners with ADHD seem to operate particularly effectively in kinaesthetic and visual situations, during which they can often maintain focus for an age/ability period of time. Opportunities to process information in mathematical/logical styles are also effective and these learners often produce concept maps which are a synthesis of a variety of techniques. The attention deficit often only seems to apply to their own work and they can learn very effectively from their keen interest in what everyone else is doing – harnessing this can empower the learners to develop their own very eclectic and effective styles of information processing and presentation.

The final key to unlocking learning is to recognise and respond to the need for movement. Brain Gym, "institutionalised fidgeting" and being asked to collect or give out materials are all ways of responding to a need to move. As always, the right to be more active must be balanced against the responsibility to do so without affecting the learning of others. The most effective management techniques focus the learner on rights, responsibilities and consequences as part of a coherent, whole class/whole school strategy.

All behaviour gets us something

The trick is to:

1. ## Work out what learners get from their behaviour

2. ## Modify the perceived reward as appropriate

Asperger's Syndrome

Asperger's Syndrome may convey the gift of concentration and focus together with an ability to pursue a line of thought or research until a conclusion is reached. It is reported that many top scientists, accountants, auditors etc have Asperger's Syndrome to some degree and it offers the opportunity to be very successful within a tight area of expertise. "Intellectual persistence" in the face of major distraction is also reported as a gift conveyed by this condition.

Like all learning differences, there are costs as well as opportunities. Asperger's Syndrome is part of the autistic spectrum and is typified by unexpected difficulties in communication and building relationships. Outside of often quite narrow areas of interest, imaginative play and creativity can be limited and learners are prone to a reliance on routines and rituals which, in extreme cases, can border on obsession. Many of the most successful mathematicians and scientists in a school may fail to achieve their potential in the arts because of a perceived weakness when it comes to being creative and "thinking out of the envelope". However when linear, step by step processing is required, linked to paying attention to the most minute details, Asperger's Syndrome is a very useful attribute.

Obsessive behaviour, typified by an insistence on sticking to routine and feelings of insecurity and panic in more fluid, open ended situations can place considerable demands on classroom management. It must be understood that any rituals which may spring from these needs are not negotiable, nor does the learner have very much choice at that time – s/he is doing what is done in order to feel safe and secure.

> The most effective management techniques focus the learner on rights, responsibilities and consequences as part of a coherent, whole class/whole school strategy

Classroom management

Teacher language seems to hold the key to effective classroom management. The language of instruction needs to be clear and unambiguous and with careful consideration given to the possibility of misunderstanding – as a rule of thumb, if language can be misinterpreted, it probably will be.

When asked to put shoes and socks on, a child refused, saying "I can't get my socks over my shoes". In another lesson the teacher said "You can't do that sum now" meaning that the lesson was nearly over and it was time to finish. Perceiving the comment to be a reflection on his mathematical ability, (as in "you can't do it because you don't know how"), the learner responded with hurt pride and verbal aggression, and was excluded.

Simple facial expressions and body language are also important – these learners are very perceptive within their areas of expertise but can be very vulnerable in relaxed "jokey" situations because they may not read the smile in the teacher's eyes or hear the smile in the voice. One boy completely misread his teacher's light-hearted instruction to "leave no stone unturned" in his search for his pencil case and got into trouble for digging up the path. Teachers with experience of working in English as an additional language will also recognise this issue – idiomatic English can be very confusing!

Given this potential for misunderstanding it is important that the teacher responds appropriately and does not over-react. Learners with Asperger's Syndrome are already vulnerable in social situations and, being acutely aware of their difficulties in understanding jokes and certain nuances, risk suffering from low self-esteem and feelings of rejection. They also risk becoming provocative victims because of problems reading body language and selecting appropriate verbal responses.

When giving instructions it is important to respond to any confusion or lack of understanding. Best advice is to repeat without re-wording, using exactly the same words, intonation and body language. Changing the words to explain can change the entire meaning for a learner with Asperger's Syndrome – the new explanation becomes a separate entity which bears little or no relation to the previous point. Of course this management technique appears to fly in the face of conventional wisdom and good practice, but it works.

It also seems to help many other learners in a classroom who appreciate a bit of "take up time". Changing the words can cause interference and/or overload in the auditory processing system so it can be a relief to be able to fill in any gaps by hearing the words again.

Asperger's Syndrome as a learning difference

Learners with Asperger's Syndrome are particularly effective when working in mathematical-logical styles involving clear guidelines and step by step processing. They tend to be linear thinkers with great powers of concentration and often have an ability to work effectively in great detail. Well-documented "obsessive" tendencies can, when properly harnessed, make these learners very effective indeed. Visual skills are sometimes very well developed and visual memory may be a real strength.

> # When giving instructions it is important to respond to any confusion or lack of understanding
>
> # Best advice is to repeat without re-wording by using exactly the same words, intonation and body language

The learning difference often confers fewer benefits in those tasks requiring empathy, imagination and open ended creativity. Also there may be a tendency to become locked into certain styles of operation – "I have my method!" – which, although clearly ineffective, is chosen because it creates a feeling of comfort and security. These learners seem to lose confidence and direction very quickly when asked to work outside of their comfort zones. An example of this would be a rigid reliance on processing information in a linear way when the task clearly calls for a mind map or similar more expansive technique.

With patience and empathy the comfort zone can be extended to embrace a variety of techniques to provide support in vulnerable areas. Creative responses to literature etc may never be a "best thing" but these learners often embrace a framework with enthusiasm and respond well to systematic approaches which scaffold their answers; they particularly seem to appreciate having a structure in which to be creative. Another effective approach is to support the development of "linear" mindmapping as a way of processing information. Once the process is explained many learners quickly appreciate the opportunities offered by a "root and branch" organisation of main points but usually revert to type with the detail which is often presented in a linear way, as bullet points or similar. I applaud this approach since it leads the learner into new areas of comfort and provides a growing repertoire of skills and techniques on which to draw.

> Learners often embrace a framework with enthusiasm and respond well to systematic approaches to scaffold their answers; they particularly seem to appreciate having a structure in which to be creative

Dyspraxia – Developmental Coordination Disorder

Dyspraxic learners usually have ability appropriate thinking and problem solving skills when given a structure in which to access and process information. They can have a "quirky" form of creativity, coming at ideas and problems from unexpected positions. The cost of being dyspraxic comes from problems with fine motor coordination, planning what to do and how to do it without having an effective structure on which to hang ideas and well- documented difficulties with personal organisation and awareness of time. Developing and sustaining relationships can also be a challenge for some who may find they become provocative victims without the strategies to deal with the situation.

Classroom Management

All learners who prefer to operate in non-traditional ways are vulnerable when expected to function in their weaker areas of competence. Dyspraxic learners seem to think as quickly as those of similar ability but experience unexpected difficulties expressing their ideas, getting them down on paper and copying off the board. They operate well through kinaesthetic and visual techniques and seem to appreciate opportunities to develop competence in mathematical/logical styles of processing.

Planning what to do and how to do it appears to be a particular area of weakness and one which merits the investment of considerable time and energy. This investment definitely seems to reap dividends, empowering learners to organise their thoughts in ability appropriate ways.

There may be a very marked discrepancy between the quality of work produced in class and that produced in a small group or 1:1 situation. Handwriting speed can also be an issue, making dyspraxic learners particularly vulnerable when the teacher relies on dictation and copying off the board in order to get through the syllabus. For some dyspraxic learners, using a lap top can make all the difference.

Responding to need without recourse to labels – a Dyslexia Friendly response

Consider a learner who has unexpected difficulties producing evidence of learning, despite ability appropriate thinking skills. S/he finds it difficult to process a sequence of instructions in one go and, when overloaded is unlikely to translate instructions into action. Because instructions rarely make sense s/he has a tendency to "tune out" when the teacher is talking and then has to rely on help from neighbours in order to keep up.

Unfortunately this learner is not very sensitive to either the power of language or the needs of others. S/he may ask for help in inappropriate ways and, persist despite obvious messages to stop, and can become isolated, bullied or victimised. Even when the instructions have been received and understood there is a tendency for weak organisational skills to make it impossible to start, especially if the task is based around auditory/linguistic processing and evidence of learning is required in sentences and paragraphs.

Watching other learners apparently working well can compound a feeling of inadequacy, leading to feelings of stress. Once stress kicks in it limits the learner to a "comfort zone only" level of response and makes it almost impossible to operate outside of the individual's learning styles and preferences.

This learner could be said to be dyslexic, dyspraxic or have Asperger's Syndrome or ADHD. S/he could also be a refugee and currently working in English as a second or additional language. On the other hand I have taught hundreds of children over the years who, despite presenting all of the signs and symptoms above and being of average ability in a number of areas, do not have a label and whose special educational need is simply to be taught the way they learn.

Teach all learners as if they are dyslexic. Use a multi-sensory, mind friendly approach, based on an understanding of learning styles and preferences to develop confidence, self-esteem and emotional intelligence

Finding the common ground

From the perspective of the busy class or subject teacher, there is no requirement for her/him to become an expert in each of the diverse learning needs because there is a great deal of common ground on which to work. One of the most effective responses to the variety of needs evident in most mainstream classrooms is to teach all learners as if they are dyslexic, using a multi-sensory, mind friendly approach based on an understanding of learning styles and preferences and the importance of developing confidence, self-esteem and emotional intelligence.

The following strategies will help:

- Find out learning styles and preferences and refer to them constantly – both in terms of pupil preference and the demands of the task.
- Point out the requirements of tasks in terms of different processing - use clear language, based on a planned sequence of instructions, giving one sound bite at a time
- Unambiguous words and phrases – let the words mean what they say
- Positive affirmative language which tells learners what to do, rather than what not to do
- Using the language of success and possibility
- Teach a range of information processing strategies to mastery and beyond so that learners can select and employ appropriate techniques
- Having learnt to work effectively within comfort zones, require learners to process information in less comfortable ways – but always from inside to out
- Where appropriate or whenever possible, use worksheets which maximise thinking and minimise writing
- Suggest alternative recording strategies and demand different ones sequentially throughout the year to encourage learners to work outside of the zone
- Invite learners to choose appropriate learning styles once the task has been set
- At the end to the task ask which styles were used
- Also ask if the choices were appropriate – a little time spent discussing choices pays off in future lessons
- Set some targets for next lesson

Top Tip

Suggest alternative recording strategies and demand different ones sequentially throughout the year to encourage learners to work outside their comfort zones

Summary

- AD(H)D, Asperger's Syndrome and Dyspraxia are discussed in terms of:

    1. Learning issues
    2. Management strategies
    3. Learning styles and preferences

- Responding to needs without recourse to labels
- Finding common ground

Chapter 9

DYSLEXIA AND REVISION
Learning how to learn

Many dyslexic learners lack confidence in their ability to learn and study. One solution is to focus less on what is to be learnt and more on how to learn it.

Most writers in the field of study skills acknowledge there to be between seven and eight stages on the road to effective learning. Learners with diverse needs, and especially those who are dyslexic, need to be supported through the stages and encouraged to develop their own strategies within the framework. An eight stage process seems to work particularly well with dyslexic learners from the age of about 7 upwards and is reported to still be effective at university level and beyond.

Stage 1 "Building the Feel-good Factor"

Any kind of learning is hard work and success often requires sacrifice and a well-developed sense of deferred gratification. A problem for the teacher can be that many learners discover, at a depressingly early age, that they cannot learn information; or rather they cannot learn it in the ways they are being taught.

In consequence the learning/revision process is unsatisfactory and unrewarding and, quite understandably, becomes marginalised and rationalised – dyslexic learners have justified leaving their revision until the night before on the grounds that "If I start too early, I will forget". This view reflects unhelpful teaching practices and also a very natural desire to do as little as possible of something which is very hard work.

To be fair to dyslexic learners, weaknesses in working memory do make them vulnerable, which is why it is so important for them to know how they learn and to work in effective ways. However the feel-good factor needs to be established in order to give a purpose for all the hard work, suffering and pain that is to follow – the learners must know why it is worthwhile for them.

> **Weaknesses in working memory can make dyslexic learners vulnerable, which is why it is so important for them to know how they learn, and to work in effective ways**
>
> **Metacognition holds the key**

1. What's in it for me?

Appealing to self-interest can be very effective, especially with older learners. Working with teenagers, it is often helpful to ask them to project themselves 5 – 10 years into the future and ask them to imagine where they see would like to be and to choose a lifestyle to go with it. The lifestyle usually involves a decent car, designer clothes and enough money to enjoy holidays, clubs and restaurants. Asking learners to close their eyes and "see" themselves in this situation is often effective.

2. Visualise success and feel proud

Another effective visualisation activity is to picture exam success, maybe imagining going to school to collect the results, seeing the grades on the slip, celebrating with friends, the pride of going home and showing parents etc, etc.

1 and 2 above are pictures which, properly accessed, can sustain a learner through some of the dark hours that inevitably occur during sustained periods of revision.

3. Keeping the engine running

Learners must be encouraged to pace themselves, to take regular breaks and to recognise that, as a revision session proceeds, the breaks need to be longer and the time spent on task reduced – otherwise the law of diminishing returns will soon come in to play. Plenty of water, exercises and healthy food will also improve learning.

Teachers need to:

- Establish the imperative for starting early

The next steps are to:

- Suggest ways of overcoming perceived memory issues

- Show how to do things differently to maximise learning

4. Starting early – making the case

The "later I start, the less time I'll have to forget" revision principle is seductive, logical and doomed to failure. While it must be treated with respect it needs to be demolished with logic and information.

I have found it helpful to do the sums with the learner – at KS4, they work out something like this:

Time spent on GCSE subjects in Years 10+11	1600+ hours
Time spent in each core subject - English, Maths etc.	400+ hours
Time spent in each option subject	240+ hours

These figures begin to set the scene and establish the enormity of the task ahead. Having softened the learners up, we now need to discuss the allocation of revision time in the run up to exams, bearing in mind the need to finish (start?) major coursework elements in a majority of subjects as well as starting to revise. Most learners suggest an hour a night, with perhaps four hours over a weekend, making a total of about nine hours each week.

The sums now look like this:

Start Date Year 11	Revision Time available for all subjects @ 9 hours/week	Revision time available per subject (n - 10)
October	300 hours	30 hours
January	180 hours	18 hours
March/April (Easter)	90 hours	9 hours

These figures are intimidating and have the potential to deter as well as motivate if not used with empathy and compassion. However they do establish the imperative for starting early. Having done this it is the teacher's responsibility to suggest ways of overcoming perceived memory issues by doing things differently in order to maximise learning.

5. Proving it works

Insanity, as defined earlier, is an occupational hazard when engaged in revision. Although revising the night before may never have been successful, many learners are wedded to the technique and believe that, if they only do it harder, they will improve. How then can the teacher intervene in the revision process?

The Dyslexia Friendly teacher begins by introducing learning activities which rely on a variety of techniques and learning styles. Mnemonics, visualisation, mental journeys, word association, mind maps etc are all techniques which merit thorough teaching and application when there is little pressure on the learners. Transforming information from one form to another, perhaps from text to bullet points to a storyboard, is particularly effective as it requires the learner to use both sides of the brain.

Teachers are also encouraged to stipulate different techniques for given tasks in order to develop competence. For example, not all learners are natural "mind-mappers". However an action research project in a primary school in Ireland found that test results after mind mapping were up to 100% higher for all children compared with other information processing techniques. It would be unfortunate for a learner to dismiss such potential gains in recall just because s/he "doesn't like mind maps".
and irresponsible of the teacher not to ensure that all learners are competent in a range of effective strategies. My response to a plaintive "I hate mind maps" is usually "You can hate them when you have learnt how to do them – then you can choose!"

Some useful activities to prove that learners can learn are as follows:

Pairs

Pairs of picture cards, playing cards or cards with subject specific pictures are placed at random face down on a surface. All players keep a close eye on proceedings as each player takes it in turn to turn over any two cards. If they are the same, s/he keeps them, if not they are turned over for the next player. Many learners with diverse needs, whose strong visual and kinaesthetic preferences convey an uncanny ability to remember where cards are, will wipe the floor with the more "academic" learners who find their traditional skills quite useless in this context.

A word to the wise, never challenge a dyslexic learner to a game of Pairs for stakes any higher that a sweet or lolly as many have the most amazing visual memories.

Kim's Game

Up to 20 items are placed in a shoe box or similar. Learners have 60 seconds or so to look at the objects and then make a list. If the items are subject specific, an added bonus can be spelling practice of key jargon words. When results are discussed there will be a natural spread of competence and success within any group and it is helpful to ask successful learners to share their strategies – and even teach them.

Helpful strategies, used unconsciously by some learners, are likely to include:

- Looking for links between objects
- Visualising position, shape, association
- Finding a rhyme or association of words

Repeating the activity, having first reminded learners of different strategies always seems to yield improved results.
If the improvements are quantified in terms of "percentage improvement" it is possible to record significant gains over a short period. Kim's game can also demonstrate the importance of review as part of the learning cycle – a key element in the 8 stages of learning. Try splitting a class into a number of groups in a memory challenge. Each group is allowed time to look and each individual writes his or her list, without collaboration. The group scores are totalled and recorded... Allow the weakest group 60 seconds just to look at the items again (encourage them to "see" as well as look) and then move the lesson on without further comment.

Later in the lesson, ask everyone to write the list again and total the group scores. It is quite likely that the weakest group after the first activity will be one of the best, if not the best this time round – and after only 60 seconds more work.

If this is the case the teacher can quantify the improvement achieved for an investment of 60 seconds, pointing out the importance of review to the revision process. This technique has rarely let me down and proves to be a very powerful way of making a key point without any nagging. It works because the truth is self evident and the learners have found it out for themselves.

Mnemonics, Word Association and Raps

Encouraging learners to experiment with these techniques following some direct teaching is likely to prove very effective. However the links and associations need to be created and owned by the learners – the imposition of the teacher's links rarely works. Linking key words together to form a story works well, especially if the story can be illustrated with a sketch or cartoon, linking both sides of the brain.
Generally the more unusual, amusing or risqué the story, the more permanent will be the learning.

What works?

- Mnemonics
- Visualisation
- Mental journeys
- Word association
- Mind maps
- Transforming information from text to bullet points to a storyboard

Just working within a learner's KAV preferences can yield remarkable results. Presenting learners with information to be learnt and offering them choices based around drawing, talking/transforming or processing in a physical way ("post-it" notes, strips of paper etc) puts responsibility firmly with them, as it should be.

Memory Tricks

- ## Looking for links between objects

- ## Visualising position, shape, association

- ## Finding a rhyme or association of words

Create a mind map

Simply one of the best ways to learn

Considerable time has been spent on supporting learners to develop and sustain a positive state of mind - learners need to be happy, secure, confident, and empowered in order to be successful. They also need strategies to pick themselves up when things start to go wrong. No matter how carefully they are prepared, they still carry with them the baggage from countless failed attempts to present evidence of their learning at an ability appropriate level. Visualising success or future lifestyle are effective strategies when the chips are down.

Ideally every revision session should begin with a re-affirmation of "Why am I doing this? What's in it for me?"

Stage 2 - Getting the facts

Getting the big picture

When faced with a question to answer or an essay to write, dyslexic learners often find it difficult to get started. Learners tell me that the difficulty is due to having too many ideas, directions and possibilities, rather than too few, so that the overwhelming number of choices leads to "paralysis by analysis". Strategies for getting the big picture allow the learner to create a map of the territory and work in both brains. This is particularly important for dyslexic learners who, because of their differently wired brains, need to access both sides in order to optimise their potential and to minimise the potential effects of any learning differences.

Trying to learn anything without first getting the big picture is like trying to do a jigsaw puzzle without the picture on the box – it can be done but it is slow and frustrating. The following technique, based around the initials TCP – QR, helps to building the big picture, whether it is a new chapter in a text book, a set of notes to revise or an exam paper:

TCP – QR. "First Aid for Reading"

The Dyslexia Friendly Strategy for Study Reading

Stages	Focus	Questions To Ask	Rationale
Stage 1 T	Title	• What does the title mean? • What is this about? • What do I know already? • Where does it fit in with other work? • What have I got to do?	Work on the title often forms a series of informed guesses regarding likely content, direction and requirements. It engages the reader's mind and begins to form the basis for "contextual guessing" when unfamiliar words are presented
Stage 2 C + P	Captions and Pictures	To be processed together. In particular scan and examine: • Anything in bold • Anything in a box • Anything with an arrow or line • Anything in bold • Any pictures, diagrams or charts • Any foot notes • Any words that leap out of the text	Captions and pictures continue the process of contextual guessing. This is a particularly important skill for dyslexic learners who tend to think faster than they read. Also some of the text will naturally catch the eye. When it does, read it.
Stage 3 Q	Questions	Read all the questions through before starting. Then ask yourself:: • What does the question mean – can I paraphrase it? • How much do I need to write – link to the marking value if appropriate? • Have I already found the answer through captions and pictures? • Do I have a rough idea of where the answer might be in the text? • Do any of the later questions provide answers for earlier ones? (They often do!) How many questions can you answer before reading the text?	Three important "Work smart rather than hard" principles need to be understood 1. Many questions can and should be answered without a thorough reading of text 2. "Free gift" answers are often available within the body of text or later questions 3. "If in doubt, leave it out" – question spot for the easy ones first, then go back if/when you have finished

Stage 4 R	Reading	"The measure of the last resort!" Skim and scan to: • Check if answers are right • Extend answers if necessary • Fill in any gaps • Identify information to tackle the high tariff answers	Learners who think faster than they read should be encouraged to make use of every bit of help to minimise any problems with information processing. Issues relating to sub text are sometimes missed – this is an opportunity cost of being empowered to answer more questions

To get the big picture try:

- Flicking through the chapter, worksheet or exam paper
- Stop and glance at anything that catches your eye:
  - Focus – on any pictures or diagrams
  - Skim/scan - any text that catches the eye
- Listing main headings or ideas

Trying to learn anything without first getting the big picture is like trying to do a jigsaw puzzle without the picture on the box

– it can be done but it is slow and frustrating

Stage 3 Chunking down – "Setting priorities to get the facts you need"

By the end of Stage 2 of the "learning how to learn" process the teacher should be working with learners who feel positive about themselves in relation to revision and who have a reasonable idea of what is expected of them. Setting priorities is the next task. Left to choose for themselves, there is a tendency for all learners, especially those who are dyslexic, to start by revising the topics they know best. This is understandable, since it is true to the important principle of starting within comfort zones and working inside out. However, pressure of time usually means that the learner needs support to develop a revision strategy based on identifying and addressing areas of weakness. A useful strategy is outlined below:

1. Choose a subject
2. Choose a completed exercise book from that subject
3. Flick through to get the big picture
4. Take each topic heading and place it in the appropriate column on the table below – starting at the bottom of each column and working up

SETTING REVISION PRIORITIES

No problems (Test me now !)	More work needed (Some knowledge)	Not a clue (Least knowledge)

Building the table up from the bottom enables the learner to create a bar chart of current strengths and weaknesses, one which should both identify areas of priority and validate the extent of current knowledge. The simple task of completing this table turned one dyslexic learner from a state of blind panic to one of quiet, if surprised confidence when he appreciated how much he really knew about a subject.

SETTING REVISION PRIORITIES

		Circulation (3)
		Homeostasis (1)
Enzymes	Digestion	Nutrition (2)
No problems (Test me Now !)	**More work needed (Some knowledge)**	**Not a clue (Least knowledge)**

Once the table is completed the next task is to look at the topics in the "Not a Clue" column and prioritise these in order of "ignorance" with a view to beginning with the topic which is the weakest of the weak. The aim is to work on all the topics in the right hand column first in order to move them into the middle column. At this point the topics need to be re-prioritised, and the same procedure followed, until all are securely in the left hand column. The process works because it breaks learning down into a series of manageable chunks.

A table, or series of tables, needs to be completed for each examination subject, regularly updated and reviewed and kept in view in the learner's bedroom or work space.

Stage 4 Learning to Remember – "Working from inside out"

A major theme of this book has been the importance of empowering learners to identify and then operate within their comfort zones for part of every lesson. It has also been suggested that it is much easier to operate in a less comfortable style of processing when beginning from a "comfortable" start. Dyslexic learners, especially those with unresolved baggage from previous failures, always seem more comfortable when moving from areas of strength to areas of perceived weakness and often seem very happy to accept fresh challenges, providing they have had a chance to "get going" within their comfort zones".

Having paid due attention to state of mind, established the big picture and chunked down to establish priorities the next stage is to identify learning styles and preferences and to develop some expertise in different ways of processing information. Ideally knowledge of individual styles and preferences will already be an everyday part of the learner's experience. This knowledge, through the process of metacognition, informs and directs information processing choices. Leaving an awareness of learning styles until Year 10 or 11 is really far too late – arguably it should be on the way at age 7 at the very least – but perhaps better late than never. 16 year old learners have actually been known to become angry and frustrated when taught how to work within their individual styles because they want to know why they were not shown before!

The principle of identifying and working within individual comfort zones has been discussed earlier. Some helpful revision techniques include:

- Highlighting new ideas, facts, information, bits to come back to
- Tick the pages that are really understood
- Big question mark when not understood – "Come back later"
- Read difficult bits out loud
- Explain to a friend
- Tape record/web cam/video main bits – play back later
- Mind map/bullet point as you go
- Make notes on strips of paper/post-its
- Visualise – either mentally or through charts and diagrams

Expecting learners to develop these skills on top of learning for major exams is asking much too much.

However, these skills can develop sequentially and naturally as part of a study skills programme designed to support and enhance learning throughout a key stage. St Richard Gwyn, a successful and very Dyslexia Friendly 11-18 comprehensive school in North Wales, made significant improvements in GCSE results through, among other things, the provision of a weekly study skills lesson for all Year 7 pupils taught by a senior member of staff. Although it was not easy to timetable and created pressure points in other curriculum areas the overall opportunity cost of teaching all pupils how to learn was perceived as being worthwhile. This approach is also valid at Key Stage 2, especially as part of a mentoring or catch up programme.

Stage 5 Explorations and Transformation

Dyslexic learners, in common with most of their peers, seem to learn best when they transform information from one form into another, say from prose into bullets and then into a mind map. This is effective because it requires the learner to "flip" between the brains, pole bridging from left brain to right and back again through a variety of tasks associated with the same material.

The table below suggests some ways in which dyslexic learners can confidently explore a subject in length. These ways have been carefully selected to minimise passive, reading based learning and to capitalise on active, mind friendly techniques which match the eclectic preferences of many dyslexic learners.

Exploring a subject in depth	
Put it in your own words – explain to a friend	An auditory/linguistic technique with an interpersonal element which relies on getting the big picture through a variety of techniques – the more the better. It can only be effective if the learner really understands and can communicate that understanding. The success criterion is the quality of the explanation

Make a mind map	Potentially involves a range of learning styles, especially if some/all of the information is on post-its or strips of paper. Visual, kinaesthetic, mathematical/logical and intra-personal preferences can be expressed. Explaining the mind map to a friend involves auditory and/or linguistic and interpersonal preferences; use of colour and drawings lock in the visual element – both will aid recall in exams.
Discuss it or just say it out loud	Turning thoughts into speech links the brains and requires conceptualisation of the learning. Recording on tape, video, or web cam is effective, especially when the recording is based on information processed in different ways – but much less effective when simply read onto tape etc.
List main points in a logical order	Initially a mathematical/logical style which becomes kinaesthetic if the information is on strips of paper etc. Pasting up the strips to form a flow chart or mind map is an effective way of pole bridging between the brains. Explaining the logic behind the chosen order serves to "lock" the learning by bringing other styles into play.
Do something physical – either with the information or while working on it	A majority of students need to manipulate information and move while learning. Just pacing the room while repeating information out loud works for many. Tapping in time as a student chants information can be effective as can learning while on an exercise machine – a music stand is useful here.

Do something physical – either with the information or while working on it (continued)	Drawing charts and diagrams with removable labels is a very effective learning technique, as is putting elements on cards and matching to make formulae. Process flow charts with removable data works well (on strips of paper etc), as does learning aspects of MFL (Modern Foreign Languages) by drawing pictures with removable labels in the target language. Making a simple model is very kinaesthetic and likely to be easy to recall in the exam room through visualisation.
Decide how it fits in to existing knowledge	Listing what is already known can offer a powerful psychological boost. Deliberately linking new knowledge to old, through pictures, word association, visualisation etc mirrors the way memory operates. Mind maps are particularly effective, as is working with a friend. Processing and matching information on strips of paper requires the learner to flip between the brains to make visual-kinaesthetic links through mathematical/logical processing techniques.
Write a song, jingle or rap to summarise your learning	Most people seem to know the words to dozens of songs without ever consciously setting out to learn them. Using rhythm and rhyme as a learning aid can be very effective – it has always been a key learning tool during early years teaching and also in MFL.

Stage 6 Learning to remember – and remembering how to learn

Learning needs to be an active process, one in which the brain is stimulated through a variety of senses (via a multi-sensory approach). The brain also seems to appreciate regular changes in the way information is processed and seems to be able to work for longer when exposed to a variety of tasks. Perhaps the least effective method of learning is just reading the information through, over and over again; only marginally less effective is copying it out. Yet both methods are often the main techniques employed by most learners – it is a wonder that anything is learnt at all. Dyslexic learners have vulnerable working memories and must, therefore, employ mind friendly techniques to overcome specific learning differences in the way they acquire and process information.

A possible reluctance to work differently has already been identified. It is generally accepted that stressed learners are less able to be creative, preferring to hide behind rote methods which, although ineffective, may feel comfortable. The mind set seems to be something like: "Just reading it through is easier than having to think about transforming it into something else. At least this way I look as though I am revising". The importance of empowering dyslexic learners to practice, gain confidence in and ultimately embrace effective, "smart" ways of revising cannot be over emphasised.

A major sticking point can be the need to extract key points from text into bullet points or whatever. Dyslexic learners, who often think faster than they read, write or spell, often begin by rejecting this style of "revision through transformation" as taking too long –especially if they have not started early enough. A powerful argument is to take them through the following steps:

- Ask them to count the number of words in a passage to be learnt.
- Work with them to extract the key points and again count the number of words.
- Having reduced, say, 250 words of prose to 50 words of key points and done the sums, the learners need to answer a simple question:
- "Which would you rather learn, 250 words, or 50 words?"

Assuming they make the appropriate choice they need to understand that the mental processes they undertook to transform text into bullets has already started the revision process and they know more now even before starting to do any formal "learning".

Some key questions for learners. During/after a revision session can you:

- Cover your notes, diagrams, bullet points, mind map etc and write/draw them from memory?
- Put information on strips of paper, muddle them up and place them in the correct order?
- Match key words with their equivalent in the target language?
- Remove labels from a diagram or chart and put them all back in the correct places?
- Visualise your mind map or flow chart and transform the information into prose?

If the answers are positive, then effective, multi-sensory revision is taking place. If the answer is a qualified "not yet" or "not quite" that is valuable in itself because it means that the learner has a clear idea of areas that need more work. The advantage of working through transformation is that it is more difficult for learners to kid themselves that they are being successful, whereas reading through or copying chunks of text does not have inbuilt indicators of success or failure.

I would suggest that the learner celebrate this partial success by referring to the Revision Priorities Table and moving the aspect from "Not a clue" to "More work needed".

SETTING REVISION PRIORITIES

	Homeostasis (Yippee!)	Circulation (3)
	Digestion	Homeostasis (1)
Enzymes		Nutrition (2)
No problems **(Test me now !)**	**More work needed** **(Some knowledge)**	**Not a clue** **(Least knowledge)**

Keeping it uppermost

The vulnerable working memory reported by many dyslexic learners can become much more efficient through constant stimulation, interaction, review opportunities and success. Anecdotal evidence suggests that active revision strategies, based on multi-sensory techniques, can empower dyslexic learners to revise as effectively as other learners and will deliver the recall of ability appropriate concepts in the exam setting. The confidence that comes with knowing the subject may also transfer to aspects of basic skills, allowing a bit more "headroom" to think about answer planning, punctuation and spelling. Presentation may also improve as the learner gets into the flow of writing – nothing spoils presentation more than constantly having to stop and think and start again.

Stage 7 Show you know – doing it for real

"Keeping the brain in gear"

It is important to emphasise both the difference between passive and active learning and the fact that the brain needs to be kept active and involved. This is especially important when responding to the specific learning differences that come with being dyslexic.

150

High sensory challenge is recognised as being important and this can be achieved by using a number of different learning methods involving a variety of learning styles within each revision session.

Putting it all together

A Dyslexia Friendly strategy could be to select from the following:

- Choose a topic from the "Not a clue" column of the revision planner

- List the main headings - perhaps write onto strips of paper or post-its

- Create a mind map, putting each heading on a short "leg" coming from the centre of the diagram (One advantage of putting headings on post-its etc is that the order can be changed without the need to re-draw)

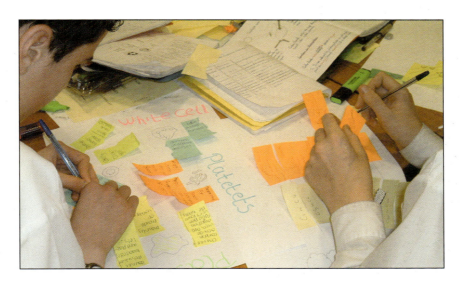

- Write key notes onto the mind map, using as few words as possible (less is definitely more in this context – the mental energy that goes into the précis of a concept helps to lock the learning)

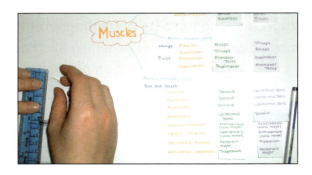

- Use colour if possible – try to link colours to concepts – e.g. using red for information relating to the "arterial" side of the circulatory system

- Explore ways of learning through the learner's comfort zone. Then, as confidence and competence increase, work from a position of security inside the zone to a less comfortable style, which usually requires flipping into a different brain – for example, by transforming bullet points (left brain) into a story board (right brain) . As before, the mental effort involved in processing information outside of the zone is often where the long term learning seems to occur

- Try re-drawing the mind map as an outline, either without words or picture or by removing the post-its etc. Then try to replace the notes or write the information into the correct places and check with the original

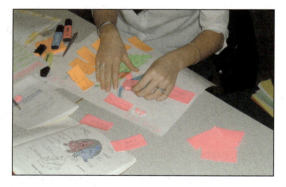

- Use the notes to create a meaningful sequence of information, perhaps as bullet points

- Turn the bullet points into a flow chart

- Explain it to someone else

- Invent a self-checking activity

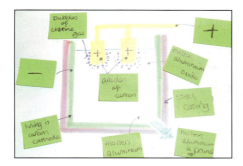

- Write a song or rap

- Create a mnemonic or "word association" story complete with cartoon

- Create a story board

Another important strategy for a learner who is trying to "show what you know" is to think up typical questions, especially those which s/he really does not want to answer. This activity helps to get the learner into the mind of the examiner and to anticipate likely questions. It also works well as part of a "study buddy" routine and is unreservedly recommended.

Building in review

Review strategies are generally recognised as being a key element in effective learning. Experience suggests the following programme to work:

1. At the end of a revision session – read over the notes, charts, mind maps etc and make aide memoirs for action in the next session
2. At the beginning of the next session – review the learning from the previous session and take any necessary action to re-learn or consolidate as required
3. At the end of each day – read over the day's revision
4. At the end of each week – read over the week's revision

Teachers who remember their early efforts to come to terms with IT in the classroom will recall how easy it was to gain competence when working with the technology on a daily basis – and how difficult it was to remember what to do after the weekend! Constant repetition, meeting challenges in different situations and finally appreciating both the big picture and the detail has enabled teachers to become very competent, after some pretty shaky starts. Also we assimilate new technology much more easily because of the confidence developed from past experience. Our dyslexic learners experience very similar highs and lows and it is possible to iron out many of the lows by supporting them to keep their revision uppermost in their minds through effective review strategies. The catch phrase is:

"Use it or lose it!"

Stage 8 Reflection – how is it going?

Just as good exam technique builds in planning time at the start of each question, good revision technique builds in time for reflection at the end of each session. Reflection is particularly important for dyslexic learners as it offers an opportunity to integrate the learning from the session into the bigger, subject based picture.

Reflection needs to be active and ideally will take a variety of multi-sensory forms. Choosing a reflection strategy which is different from the learning strategy can be particularly effective. Whatever strategy is used, five questions need to be addressed. They are:

1. What have I learnt today?

2. What has been successful/unsuccessful?

3. Can I move anything into another column on my revision planner?

4. Where are the gaps and how can I fill them?

5. Have I been using the appropriate learning styles for the task?

Reflection has the potential to put the learner in charge of the learning process. If things are not going well, a change of learning style is indicated. Although this may involve going outside of the comfort zone in order to make progress, the effort is usually worth while and explains why it is so important to build up a repertoire of learning styles and strategies.

Summary

- Learning how to learn
- The feel-good factor
- Setting revision priorities
- Getting the facts
- Chunking down
- Learning to remember (1)
- Exploration and transformation
- Learning to remember (2)
- Show you know
- Reflection

Chapter 10

MATHS AS A SPECIFIC LEARNING DIFFERENCE

Maths has a language all of its own. In consequence Dyslexia Friendly teachers will be able to make good use of EAL skills and techniques to develop understanding. The need for numeracy across the curriculum makes it essential that all teachers have an understanding of the issues for dyslexic learners and are able to draw on a repertoire of "hot tips" to overcome or minimise likely problems. Many of the difficulties seem to result from:

- A failure to develop the language of mathematics
- A lack of consistency regarding the language used
- The way techniques are taught

Also many of the literacy acquisition problems facing dyslexic and EAL learners – laterality, perceptual issues, sequencing, processing information and limited working memory – all impinge upon the acquisition of numeracy. In consequence it is essential that the translation to and from the two languages is explicitly taught and sequentially reinforced – in a Dyslexia Friendly school all contact staff will be aware that no learning can be taken for granted, not even something apparently successfully taught only minutes ago.

Best practice across the curriculum in mainstream settings is to use language which supports the learner to recognise familiar situations within the English language. Just as with literacy, the acquisition of numeracy relies on working from the known to the unknown – there is no point charging ahead with new concepts until the basics are in place. Also the Dyslexia Friendly school will implement policy and practice to allow time for teachers to re-visit early concepts and skills, permitting learners to work from their comfort zones and start from inside out. Eminent writers in the field, such as Chinn and Sharma, emphasise the importance of understanding the words and of introducing a standard and commonly understood mathematical language based on an agreed vocabulary. This is particularly important for learners with vulnerable working memories. Links can be seen with learners with Asperger Syndrome. Once again it is essential that the words mean what the words mean –any ambiguity has the potential to cause confusion, frustration, stress and a loss of automaticity.

Oral strategies like "pair-share" and barrier games are equally valuable in Maths, supporting learners to articulate concepts, procedures and strategies before committing to paper. Getting it down on paper is particularly threatening because of the perceived black and white nature of mathematical processing.

For issues regarding confusion with place value + choosing the right process try:

- Using graph paper to support accurate setting out of sums in all subjects
- Keeping it kinaesthetic – hands on place value activities will support development of the concept
- Keeping it real and go for "ball park figures" – rounding up and rounding down to get a "guesstimate" that fits. Then go back and look at place values and process
- Ensuring new information links with previous knowledge

For issues with remembering mathematical symbols try:

- Using the language of maths at every opportunity to link words and symbols
- Precision teaching – short quizzes to over-learn the relationship between symbol and process
- Ensuring new information links with previous knowledge – essential to work from inside out
- Going back to re-learn/re-emphasis early concepts and skills
- Frameworking the maths to ensure that the acquisition of important numerical concepts in, say, History or Science do not founder on the mechanics of the sums

For issues with reversals try:

- Being prepared for reversals – likely to be a constant issue for dyslexic learners

- Marking for process – insist working is shown to enable the teacher to back track. Learner resistance to showing the working can be countered by unpacking the marking process and demonstrating:

  1. How many marks are available for a well-worked answer which is wrong
  2. How reversed number strings can be right if the working gives a clue

For issues with learning tables try:

- Being gentle, as tables are likely to be a nightmare for many dyslexic learners – the learning process targets many typical areas of weakness
- Investing time in number bonds and the relationship between numbers – precision teaching gives an effective return for the time invested
- Looking for "free gifts" – 3x6 gives the learner 6x3

For issues with mental maths try:

- Taking the pressure off and being gentle!
- Ensuring the right to pass is in place
- Considering working a small group separately with another adult or a peer to lead the activity
- Wherever possible, using pair/share activities
- Giving take up time
- Giving hands on materials to support thinking

For issues with reading the question try:

- Over learning the language – and be prepared to do it again and again. "Taught is learnt" is not a mantra for a Dyslexia Friendly school
- Reinforcing key words and phrases with flash cards, precision teaching etc
- Explaining to a partner - pair/share activities work well

- Transforming the question into a mind map or story board – answering the "who, what, why, where, when, how" questions will support comprehension
- Going for guesstimates – require learners to articulate and justify their ball park figure and reduce stress by asking for an answer with a wide "plus or minus" range

For issues with telling the time try:

- Going digital – for simplicity and expediency
- Practicing the language – peer tutoring and precision teaching
- Giving take up time
- Marginalising the importance until the learner is clearly ready

A theme of this book is the way that teaching and learning problems and solutions are often generic – there is a common thread of approaches and responses that can meet most needs in most situations. The table below suggests generic approaches for numeracy and literacy, many of which will also transfer to ESL (English as a Second Language) situations.

Numeracy and Literacy – matching needs and responses	
Mathematical Needs and Responses	**Literacy Needs and Responses**
• When a pupil is stuck, give "instant answers" and encourage to repeat while the teacher/TA is watching	• Give spellings when a learner is in the flow of writing. Mark "on the hoof" to reinforce good practice
• Test papers and worksheets need to be uncluttered, with room for working out	• Worksheets need to minimise writing and maximise thinking – uncluttered and "obvious"

- Avoid testing too much at once – target the testing to currently taught work. If you want to test something else, revise it first – please do not "spring it" on the learners

- Clear links with spelling tests. Avoid the tyranny of a jumble of words requiring the assimilation of a variety of spelling rules

- Make sure assessments test what has actually been taught and learnt, rather than a "wish list". Also be aware that many tests actually assess reading and writing skills rather than understanding of concepts and process

- 1:1 assessments (with teacher, TA or buddy) will be a more accurate reflection of learning (and the effectiveness of teaching). The willingness to accept evidence of learning in a variety of forms typifies a Dyslexia Friendly teacher

- Both aspects benefit from being taught in as multi-sensory a way as possible. Dyslexia Friendly spelling techniques – the sand tray, visualisation, sky writing etc – while saying it out loud are equally effective with the language and processes of Maths. Chanting procedures while doing Brain Gym is also well worth the effort and apparent risk of disruption – in reality the learners appreciate the opportunity to move and soon link successful learning with the physical activity.

Using Technology

IT can offer dyslexic learners another way to show what they know while waiting to develop their literacy skills. The key factor will be access to a desk top or lap top computer whenever required. There is a mistaken view that a laptop is a panacea for all dyslexic ills, especially at secondary level; for every learner who thrives on the use of technology, there is usually another one who much prefers more traditional means of recording and processing information. Problems with spell checks are well-documented; less well documented are issues like being able to get a paper copy on demand (it is very difficult to tick a computer screen) and storing printed information can be a major challenge.

The multi-sensory nature of typing is a boon to many, but other learners find the co-coordinational skills very difficult to acquire, a problem which can compound difficulties with information processing and spelling. Keying in complex, polysyllabic words can place particular demands on sequential memory.

One potentially valuable piece of technology is Speech Recognition Software (SR). The learner speaks into the computer and the computer writes what is said.
The British Dyslexia Association has produced a good bulletin on SR which looks at opportunities and costs. A summary is quoted below:

Opportunities

- The learner speaks and the words appear on screen, correctly spelt, needing less well-developed keyboard skills
- Some systems have a playback facility which supports a vulnerable short term memory and helps with proof reading
- Some learners have found SR liberating and report improvements in spelling and reading because they are always reading their own correctly spelt words
- A success rate of 90-98% is claimed. Spelling 9 words out of 10 may be an improvement over typing or writing
- Provided that SR is the learner's usual way of working, exam boards may allow its use
- It can be a life skill which will transfer to college, university and beyond
- Success depends on the development of effective information processing skills and places an imperative on the development of planning techniques, especially mind mapping
- The software is priced from about £50 upwards

Costs

- A powerful modern computer is recommended and desktops generally seem to work better than laptops

- A good quality microphone is essential and careful attention needs to be paid to the position of the microphone throughout a session
- The software has to be trained to the learner's voice - this can be a major sticking point for those with strong regional accents or EAL
- Boys may need to retrain after puberty
- Dictation skills need to be developed, together with effective planning and information processing techniques. These must be taught, learnt and used
- Although all words may be spelt correctly, proof reading may be more of a challenge – it is much harder to spot the "wrong" word when it is correctly spelt

A growing number of schools are finding software based planning programmes to be effective with their dyslexic learners. Inspiration (including Kidspiration) and Mind Genius are two useful mind mapping programmes which can be used to complement SR technology.

Learners who prefer to use a keyboard may find Wordbar (from the Clicker suite by Crick) very useful indeed. It is a toolbar, containing teacher/learner prepared words and phrases which sits along the bottom of the screen. The appropriate word and phrases are clicked to send them to the screen and integrate into the text being typed. It works across the curriculum and has an EFL application – indeed the only limitation is teacher time and imagination.

Summary

- Using technology – opportunities and costs
- Numeracy and literacy – matching needs and responses

Chapter 11

DYSLEXIA AND EAL
Mind friendly solutions for Dyslexia as a second language

The key issues are identification and response, just as with native speakers of English. However, learners with EAL require a different perspective and there is a need to separate the expected general language and skill acquisition issues caused by a current lack of language proficiency from the unexpected issues which are likely to be present in the first language as well.

While running a study skills course with learners from the international community in Hungary I was struck by the similarities between their problems with information acquisition and processing when operating in English and those of native English speakers who were dyslexic.

The similarities included:

- A tendency to lose the thread when processing information - key bits of information would get lost
- Skill overload – the learners could either write fluently or spell/punctuate accurately in their second language (L2), but rarely both at the same time
- Vulnerable sequencing skills – especially when required to perform reasonably lengthy step by step processing
- Short term memory lapses
- Word finding – especially under pressure of time or teacher scrutiny
- Speed of processing – especially the development of automaticity

The similarities became more marked as I refined my teaching in response to their needs.

These mainly non-dyslexic learners, with a disparate range of experience in English as an additional language worked best when:

- Their learning preferences were identified and they were shown how to work effectively within their comfort zones
- The learners were provided with a repertoire of information accessing and processing techniques and given time so that they could operate confidently and automatically within their chosen styles and techniques
- They were taught a range of memory techniques and provided with over-learning opportunities
- Sound/symbol correspondence was checked using chunking strategies, clapping syllables and the "Make and Break" multi-sensory spelling technique was taught to mastery
- Multi-sensory information processing techniques, based around the use of colour, strips of paper/post-its and mind mapping, were taught and consolidated
- Good practice was modelled at every opportunity when the teacher composed and wrote text
- Frameworks were used to scaffold writing

The techniques above were developed in response to learner need and it is sobering to reflect that, by allowing my teaching to be learner driven, I found myself automatically teaching in a Dyslexia Friendly way - all the strategies used were part of my normal "Dyslexia repertoire".

As the course developed I began to notice variations in the way some learners were responding. Some were picking up the skills and running with them, modifying them to suit their preferences and becoming increasingly happy to work outside of their comfort zones. Others were less confident and slower to develop certain skills. They also much preferred to operate within areas of strength and became stressed when over faced. Familiarity with English did not seem to be the determining factor - the differences could not be put down to linguistic competence. Also these learners were able to express ideas and concepts effectively in both their own language (L1) and English (L2). What seemed to be happening was that some learners were experiencing an "unexpected difficulty" when it came to acquiring and processing information and then presenting it in different forms – they could be dyslexic.

Assessment "on the hoof" is a well tried and tested teaching technique and it became possible to develop a hypothesis that language acquisition issues for EAL learners may well be due to dyslexia if:

- Unexpected difficulties in skill acquisition in L2 had already been identified
- Adequate opportunity to learn had been given
- Appropriate teaching had taken place and could be seen to be effective with learners from a very similar linguistic background
- The learners were happy to work within their comfort zones but very quickly became overloaded when asked to move "outside"
- Crucially, similar learning differences were evident when operating in L1

A pragmatic rule of thumb for identifying specific issues for Dyslexia and EAL seems to be a combination of the following:

- An individual learner's level of skill acquisition and conceptual development in L1
- Performance in L1 in comparison with L2
- Progress in L2 benchmarked against the progress of other learners in the group

Finding ways of assessing linguistic competence in L1 is likely to be very important when faced with apparently unexpected difficulties. Weak phonological skills in L1 will almost inevitably transfer negatively to L2; reading skills above basic level at L1 may well transfer positively to L2.

Also there seems to be a well-established cross language transfer from L1 phonological skills to L2 word reading. Therefore the involvement of community professionals to establish the level of L1 competence seems to be indicated before considering further assessment and certainly before involving an educational psychologist.

Discussions with the family are not always easy to achieve, especially during school hours. Teachers report some success by visiting the home at the weekend or in the evening, especially when accompanied by a member of the community.

Careful questioning in L1 can establish the incidence of the following indicators:

- Phonological errors
- Visual errors
- Working memory issues
- Family history
- Clumsiness and poor balance
- Poor sequencing

If these problems are already evident in the L1 environment and can be bench marked against other well established skills and competencies within the same environment then we may well be looking at problems at L2 being due to specific learning differences.

A strategy for response and support

- Teach all EAL learners as if they are dyslexic
- Establish their learning styles and preferences and work from inside out
- Be aware of unexpected difficulties in skill acquisition in relation to others in the same group
- Base teaching and learning around kinaesthetic, visual and mathematical-logical preferences while encouraging learners to go beyond these whenever they perceive the need or opportunity
- Establish a high challenge, low stress, learning environment based around opportunities for learners to present work in a variety of forms
- Get into the community to establish level of competence at L1

If one or two learners continue to struggle while the rest flourish it is likely that additional help and support will be required, in which case, refer to the SENCO.

Summary

- Identifying similarities between EAL and Dyslexia
- Effective strategies for EAL
- Identifying unexpected difficulties within an EAL background
- Generic support strategies for Dyslexia and EAL

Chapter 12

A TOOLKIT FOR THE DYSLEXIA FRIENDLY CLASSROOM

Identification and response in mainstream settings

Section 1 – Dyslexia at the chalk face "Who, What, why, where, When"

This section offers guidance and support for non specialist teachers in their daily contact with dyslexic learners. Answers are provided to common questions and there is a checklist of common concerns which is linked to concrete suggestions for classroom based responses.

Who is dyslexic – what do I look out for?

About 10% of pupils in our schools experience "unexpected difficulties" in acquiring certain basic skills. The key word is "unexpected": such children are usually able to think and/or talk about a topic as well as their peers – that is to say at an ability appropriate level. It is when they come to work independently (reading it, writing it etc) that unexpected problems often occur for about 3 pupils in every classroom in every school in Liverpool, in the North West across the UK and beyond. Does this description fit any children you teach?

What is Dyslexia?

A useful working definition is:

> "An unexpected difficulty in acquiring basic skills, despite adequate opportunity for learning and ability appropriate strengths in other areas"

Dyslexia is also known as one of the "specific learning difficulties" which prevent children from learning at an ability appropriate level.

So a dyslexic pupil will demonstrate understanding of the theme, topic and/or concept during group work, through oracy, etc. yet will display **unexpected problems** when it comes to getting it down on paper.

The definition also refers to "**adequate opportunity**." Some pupils "won't" read, write, whatever – they have the skills, but choose not to use them. Dyslexic pupils "can't" do some things because certain skills just are not available yet, despite apparently having been taught them. "Taught is learnt" is a dangerous belief for any child; it is doubly dangerous for children with specific learning difficulties.

What about ESL as a "lack of adequate opportunity"? Pupils for whom English is a second or additional language have difficulties through a current lack of opportunity. In fact, not only do they share many problems with their dyslexic peers, but the solutions are very similar. The "Dyslexia Friendly" classroom works for ESL as well.

> # Best practice guide is to teach all pupils, as if they are dyslexic!

Why bother to change for 10% of the class, - what about the other 90%?

Strategies for addressing Dyslexia in mainstream settings usually make teaching and learning more effective for all pupils, including the more able and talented. Regardless of learning need, a majority of pupils seem to make better progress, stay on task for longer and achieve better results when taught in a Dyslexia Friendly way.

Fine-tuning teaching for 10% seems to make the management of learning and behaviour more effective for all because, by and large, "progressing kids are happy kids". Experience also suggests that happier children have happier parents and do better in SATs, GCSE etc. Creating a Dyslexia Friendly approach has the potential to be a win-win situation.

Where does all this "different" stuff take place?

Dyslexia Friendly schools have Dyslexia Friendly classrooms, run by Dyslexia Friendly teachers. In other words, the approach pervades all aspects of teaching and learning all of the time. Fortunately, it seems to work for a majority of pupils. If we teach dyslexic children as if they are slow learners, they learn very little; if we teach slow learners as if they are dyslexic, they learn to achieve at an ability appropriate level The effectiveness of "classroom action" is a key indicator of the effectiveness of the school's inclusion policy as well as a measure of dyslexia friendliness.

Most children with any identified learning needs, at School Action, School Action Plus or with a Statement, spend a majority of their time in the mainstream class – usually 90+% of their time in school is spent being taught in mainstream settings.

Most of us also work daily with children who have ADHD, Autistic Spectrum Disorders, EBD, Dyspraxia, MLD and Speech and Language issues. In consequence, most of the "special education" has to take place in the classroom. This is why the UK Code of Practice, supported by OFSTED, states that all teachers are teachers of children with special educational needs. Techniques used to include dyslexic children are also effective across this spectrum of diverse needs.

When should "Dyslexia Friendly" teaching occur?

The simple answer is "all the time, every time, with everybody".

The strategies outlined next are grounded in the psychology of leaning and are part of the accelerated learning approach. They work with pupils who are Dyslexic, with those with more diverse needs and, in fact, for all learners in every class.

The next section deals with what to look out for and what to do about it.

INDICATORS OF DYSLEXIA/SPLD

- looking for a pattern of strengths and weaknesses -

A pragmatic indicator is to look for pupils who experience **unexpected difficulties in light of their other strengths and abilities.**

It is also important to view this pattern in relation to ability because Dyslexia occurs across a wide range of ability. Therefore it is helpful to identify specific weaknesses in skill acquisition in relation to "ability appropriate" performance in other areas.

USING A CHECKLIST

Care needs to be taken when using a checklist. Checklists are indicators of strengths and weaknesses not assessment tools. What it should do is to trigger some fine-tuning of teaching and learning in the mainstream classroom. A pupil with a persistent clustering of indicators will almost certainly benefit from being taught in a Dyslexia Friendly way. Many children will make progress following a change of approach. Those that do not may require further intervention, perhaps in the form of School Action.

Under no circumstances should any checklist be used to say a child "is" dyslexic.

> # Checklists are indicators of strengths and weaknesses not assessment tools.
>
> # Checklists should not be used to identify a child who is Dyslexic!

Accentuating the Positive

STRENGTHS	Noted	Action
Often **imaginative and creative, lateral thinker**, original solutions to problems.		
May be **skilful** in design and construction, IT etc. Often **"knows" how things work** without reading instructions, manuals etc.		
May be very **visual**, often "thinks in pictures", sometimes artistic		
Often sociable and **verbally able**		
May **enjoy drama, sport (often individual activities)**		
Ability appropriate interest in and knowledge of science, technology, current affairs etc		

Summary

It is not all doom and gloom. Dyslexia often conveys gifts in terms of certain strengths and abilities.

A very Dyslexia Friendly approach is to:

1. Find out what children are good at
2. Give them the chance to do more of it
3. Catch them doing it right

Chapter 13

RESPONDING TO NEEDS THROUGH CLASSROOM ACTION

The tables below list various issues which may affect learning. Each issue at Key Stage 1-4 has a reference which links to intervention strategies selected for their ease of application in mainstream settings. The strategies are intended to be as inclusive as possible, supporting teachers to select interventions which will fit unobtrusively into the normal delivery of the lesson.

PRE-SCHOOL (may also be evident throughout the Key Stages)

N.B. Many nursery nurses are already identifying "unexpected difficulties" at this stage. For example, they may notice children who have problems with buttons, laces etc yet show great skill with Duplo, Sticklebricks and other coordinational activities.

Issues	Noted	Action
Speech – may be slow to develop		
Rhyme – may be insensitive to rhyme/have difficulty learning nursery rhymes, jingles etc		
Name finding – problems even with known objects		
Remembering instructions – easily overloaded		
Walks early – **may not have crawled**		
Dressing skills – problems with buttons, laces etc		
Motor control – problems with throwing, catching, kicking		
"Good days and bad days" – for no obvious reason		

KEY STAGES 1-4

1. GENERAL BEHAVIOURS	Noted	Action
1.1 **General lack of confidence** – may have well-developed avoidance strategies		
1.2 **Self esteem** – lacks confidence, "rubbishes" skills/abilities		
1.3 **Concentration** – often poor, unless the child has chosen the task		
1.4 **Distractible** – paying attention to everything, but often focussing on very little		
1.5 **Disorganised** – problems organising work and self (wrong books, kit, materials)		
1.6 **Stamina** – tires easily		
1.6 **Over-reaction to failure** – may choose not to try rather than risk failure or over-react with emotional outbursts		
1.8 **Good days and bad days** for no apparent reason		
1.9 **Poor memory** – days of the week, weeks in the year, anything in a sequence, anything with more than 1-2 parts		
1.10 **Laterality** – persistent problems with left and right		

CLASSROOM STRATEGIES

1. General Behaviours

1.1/2 – General lack of confidence and low self-esteem

"We have no control over the state in which learners arrive at our lesson. We have total control over our response". Mike Hughes

- To set a pupil up to succeed:
    - Find out what they are good at and give them the opportunity to do more of it
    - Give them a taste of success

- Communicate that it is "ok to be dyslexic" and that "I like you the way you are"
- Move away from the National Curriculum for a while to guarantee success
- Set individual targets that are easy to achieve/impossible to miss – stay within comfort zones and aim for an "error free" situation at first
- Mark all the words spelt correctly and give a score out of words written
- Set up to succeed using learning styles and preferences
- Use the language of success:
  - "I know you can (avoid going on to say "if you try harder!")
  - "As soon as you have finished that bit you can ...."
  - "This is tricky at the moment but I will give you all the help you need to do a good ....."
  - "Great effort – you are much closer to the right answer now"
- And, just for a change try:
  - "I bet you can't..." when you know very well they can and will!
  - Link it to a reward if appropriate
  - Encourage risk taking
- Use the language of possibility – following complaints that work is too hard/boring etc:
  - Initially agree with the learner
  - Re-frame as " a bit tricky just now," or "it gets more interesting when this bit is out of the way"
  - "Which bit can't you do yet?"
  - "Which bit didn't I explain well enough?"
  - "If I write/do the first bit, can you carry on?"
  - Refer to the learner's strengths

1.3 Concentration

- Is it a "can't" or a "won't"? Compare concentration and focus between a set task and one of the learner's choosing – if there is a marked difference in favour of the personal task it may reflect a learning preference issue

- Compare attention when 1:1/small group with performance in class – it may be "sensory overload" caused by an inability to filter out extraneous noise and select the appropriate messages
- Work within comfort zones as much as possible
- Highlight key information – e.g. process sign in Maths
- Fewer words – more visual examples
- Increase amount of eye contact
- Monitor frequently for understanding
- Utilise a great deal of colour, movement and graphics
- Limit the number of concepts introduced at one time
- Secure attention before giving instructions
- Insist on a "physical" acknowledgement of attention when giving instructions – "Lift your head and look at me"
- Give instructions one bite at a time – warn learner that s/he may be asked to repeat to teacher, TA or buddy
- Use positive, affirmative language – say what is wanted rather than what is not wanted
- Make sure key information for action is in the first sound bite
- Discuss with SENCO if this good practice fails to work with one learner, despite being effective with others

1.4/5 – Distractible/disorganised

- Clarity of expectations – expressed in positive language: "Do..." rather than "Don't..."
- Cueing, prompting and reminders to re-establish focus
  - "That looks good. Read that bit to me please"
  - "What are you going to do next?"
  - "What have we got to do next?"
  - "Can you remember what I said about....? Well done. Now please will you....."
- Active learning – maintain a high level of kinaesthetic learning, particularly in Years 5+6 and especially at Key Stages 3+4
- Offer help with organisation and study skills
- Predictable schedules and routines
- Choices
- Extra time to process and/or perform tasks

- Manage the learner:
  - Elicit eye contact and/or touch learner before giving verbal commands (teacher's judgement re: appropriateness of using touch)
  - Increase teacher proximity to learner
  - Vary tone of voice – verbal style
  - Present at a snappy, lively pace, but be gracious when asked to repeat/recap
  - "Less is more" – especially when giving instructions so be sure to "think then say"
  - Give take up time after giving instructions
- Small steps – chunk activities/delivery for plenty of beginnings and ends – not too much in the middle
- Organise the learner through:
  - Teacher/aide/buddy recording assignments
  - End-of-day clarification of assignments/reminders to learner
  - End-of-day check by teacher/aide for expected books/materials to take home
- Use positive affirmative language – see 1.3/4 above
- Work by numbers – one chunk at a time
- Support by developing organizational strategies – list in Planner, good parental links
- Ask family to share any strategies that work at home
- Encourage learner to "come clean" when things are left at home, rather than wait until a crisis develops
- Make what is required absolutely clear and unambiguous
- Try setting up a large plastic place mat with marked spaces for pen, pencil, ruler rubber etc so that everything is laid out and ready for use. Also consider using tape to mark the optimum angle for the exercise book to facilitate comfortable writing. This is working well in a number of schools as part of a whole class strategy
- Involve peers
- Be prepared for regular disappointment and frustration – often one step forward and several back, especially on dyslexic days

1.6 Tires easily

- Dyslexic learners may need to work up to five times harder than their peers just to keep up, so be patient and supportive
- Being dyslexic is often like working in another language – information needs to be received accurately, processed so that it makes sense and then re-processed in order to present the information as stipulated by the task – so provide a framework, plan or series of sentence starters
- Compare performance and stamina on a learner selected task – if there is a marked difference it may be a "choosing issue" related to learning styles and preferences. Try changing the learning styles in use or offer more choice regarding the nature of evidence required
- Chunk tasks and activities
- Offer frequent "time out" opportunities
- Challenge endurance through targets
- Discuss with family and SENCO

1.7 Good days and bad days

Offer sympathy and understanding. "Walk the talk" by:

- Using the language of possibility and success
- Set realistic targets
- Set up to succeed, especially on bad days
- Offer choices
- Be relaxed about it

1.8   Over-reaction to failure

- Avoid putting pupils on the spot
- Try creating small group/1:1 situations for quick-fire mental activities
- Try generating group questions. These can be in the form," Our group would like to know…."
- Use immediate, frequent and positive feedback – "I really like the way you….."

- Mark for success – identify the good points and acknowledge "development/improvement points" – "This could be even better if...."
- Use the word "quiz" instead of "test"
- Set appropriate pass marks – build in the opportunity to make "safe" mistakes by asking for 6/10 rather than 10/10
- This is your chance to show how much you have learnt about this topic and you have some choices about how to do it You can:
  - Write a paragraph
  - Draw a labelled diagram
  - Do a mind map/story board/flow chart
  - Tell your Teaching and Learning Assistant/Buddy
  - Choose your own way to do the task

1.9 Poor memory

- Categorise and chunk information
- One bite at a time
- Link to earlier knowledge information – encourage learner to make links
- Look for associations:
  - Visual – pattern, shape, colour, ridiculous pictures
  - Conceptual – grouping, pattern
  - Auditory – sound, rhyme, rhythm
  - Acronyms – DEAR = "Drop everything and read"
  - Silly sentences /Mnemonics – "Big elephants can always understand small elephants"
- Teach and practice visualisation – "Try writing a word on your eyelids. Can you see it? Tell me the letters in reverse order"
- Ask pupil to repeat instructions/paraphrase before starting - to teacher/aide/buddy
- Provide a list of activities for the learner to tick off as s/he completes
- Provide hard copies of material from projectors and black or white boards, etc.

1.10 Laterality

- It really is no big deal – laugh with the child
- Ask others teachers to admit to their laterality problems – especially when giving/following directions when driving

- Visual clues – watch on right hand tells the right time
- Create practice opportunities – "I bet you can't point to my left hand with your right hand"

2. READING

Issue	Noted	Action
2.1 Difficulties with **sound/symbol correspondence** – knowing what sounds letters make. May know most, but some correspondence problems are persistent		
2.2 **Phonological skills** – learning nursery rhymes/jingles, identifying initial/medial/final sounds, hearing/tapping syllables, blending sounds		
2.3 **Laterality and direction** – unsure of which hand to use to write, eat etc. Also unsure of left and right. Problems giving/listening to directions		
2.4 **Unexpected problems acquiring high frequency words** – especially in light of ability appropriate spoken vocabulary. May acquire some words but be "blocked" on others, despite persistent support		
2.5 **Inconsistent** – may read a word correctly on one line but not on next		
2.6 **Slow, hesitant reader** – often well-developed avoidance strategies		
2.7 **Gets tired easily** – less accurate reading at the end of the session/day.		
2.8 **Loses place without guide** (ruler/finger). May miss out/add words, jump forward or back to another line. May re-read lines/paragraphs without realising		
2.9 **Finds it difficult to skim/scan**. May read passage accurately but have unexpected difficulties identifying main ideas and/or extracting detail		

2.1 Difficulties with sound/symbol correspondence

- Relax – both teachers and learners. Do not let it become an issue under any circumstances because things will improve when the learner is ready. When is that? When it happens!
- Go kinaesthetic – make sure magnetic letters and small boards or wooden letters etc are immediately available (especially at KS3+4

– older learners appreciate this approach becoming the house style in order to minimise feelings of stigmatisation. If everyone does it then it is ok to do it if you are dyslexic

- Use precision teaching techniques – quick tests before school, at lunch time and to take home for pupils to practice a restricted number of sounds/symbols and chart their own progress
- If the above are not helping, mention to SENCO

2.2 Weak phonological skills

- Go kinaesthetic – Smart Kids have some superb games and magnetic boards/letters work well. In addition try cutting up rhymes and jungles into words and/or phrases to be rebuilt by the learner (remember Breakthrough to Literacy?) These are very appropriate activities to use in place of some of the morale sapping elements of Literacy Hour. Feel free to teach the child rather than cover the curriculum!
- Work from the learner's rhyming preferences – pop songs/raps/ silly rhymes etc. Haiku is good for syllables and rhythm and effective rap relies on rhythm and rhyme.
- If the above are not helping, mention to SENCO

2.3 Laterality and direction

Research among teachers attending my presentations suggests that many highly intelligent and well-qualified professionals do not have automaticity with regard to left and right, so it does not need to be an issue.

- Visual clues can help – wearing a watch on the right hand for "right time"
- Get the learner to devise tricks, mnemonics, pictures, rhymes etc. A player from a rival football team who plays on the left should be "left back in the changing room". Which is the "right side" for a named member of a boy/girl band to stand? The key is to support learners to come up with meaningful strategies of their own
- Barrier games are very effective for giving/listening to instructions – they have application in all subjects, at all ages and at all levels of ability. Also they are especially effective at KS3

and 4 as "catch up" practice for older learners who are "hungry to improve" and appreciate working in a different way

- If the above are not helping, mention to SENCO

2.4 Unexpected problems acquiring high frequency words

- A classic dyslexic tendency. Pay attention to the learner's emotional needs by not making an issue of the small words – they are important, but not at the expense of the feel-good factor
- If in doubt – ignore them. Justify this approach through target marking but make sure parents understand what is happening and why!
- Move on to phonically regular polysyllabic words – this often helps to reinforce high frequency words
- If the above are not helping, mention to SENCO

2.5 Inconsistent – may read a word correctly on one line but not on the next

- Another classic dyslexic tendency – arguably a key indicator of specific learning issues and caused, in part, by memory issues. Words read correctly earlier on the page can present as a completely different word further on
- Relax – both teachers and learners. Do not let it become an issue under any circumstances
- Although it will improve as the learner achieves readiness it is always likely to surface under pressure
- Encourage the use of context – encourage the learner to say "blank" or "blankety blank" when s/he comes to a problem word and read to the end of the sentence
- Teacher/Assistant/Buddy reads the sentence, missing out the problem word
- Ask the learner to say the letter names of the problem word – this often seems to work. Saying letter sounds does not seem to be as effective. If the above are not helping, mention to SENCO

2.6 Slow, hesitant reader – may avoid reading

- All behaviour gets us something. We need to find the message in the learner's response to reading to determine if the reluctance is a "can't or won't" issue
- Relax – both teachers and learners. Do not let it become an issue under any circumstances
- Never, under any circumstances, demand that the learner reads out loud to the rest of the group – invite to read but ensure that the right to pass is available. (Ironically it is often the slowest, most hesitant readers who volunteer – if so, ask them for one or two lines only or set them up with a buddy to "pair read" the piece)
- Set up buddies to pair read for comprehension activities etc – information on tape/disc with the learner reading out loud from a transcript can work well across the curriculum. Study buddies/older learners may enjoy doing the taping as part of community service
- On a 1:1 basis try using a pointer to point to a word while the learner is reading the one before and increase the pressure to look beyond the target word
- If the above are not helping, mention to SENCO

2.7/8   Gets tired easily/loses place without a guide

- Make guides available to all pupils and encourage their use by all pupils for certain tasks – many will benefit, especially older pupils
- It helps if the teacher regularly models the use of a guide when reading
- Present material on pastel shades of paper – buff seems particularly good
- Make coloured overlays to put over page – allow reader to choose the colour
- Put pages from text books in transparent wallets of appropriate colours – they need to be open on two sides - readily available from stationary suppliers etc
- Consider photocopying national exam papers on to preferred paper colours
- Check the lights – does s/he read better/have more stamina with the lights off? If so, check lights for flicker and glare
- If the above are not helping, mention to SENCO

2.9 Skimming/scanning difficulties

- Check readability of passage – it may be too hard
- Hear the learner read – more than 2 mistakes per 10 words means the passage is too hard, indicating the need to differentiate the reading
- Play "I bet you can't find the word ????? in this line/in this paragraph" and "Put your finger on this word/phrase……" on a regular basis, especially in History, Science, Maths etc, etc. Initially teachers may need to limit the area to be scanned (e.g. in first paragraph, top half of page etc) but competence improves rapidly
- Use TCP-QR
- Be aware of the remarkable ability of some pupils with EAL to read with great fluency and accuracy but with minimal comprehension. Teachers are advised to ask questions like "So what does this mean? How does this take us forward? What has happened – what will happen next?" throughout the reading sequence
- If the above are not helping, mention to SENCO/EAL coordinator

3. SPELLING

3.1	**Severe and persistent difficulties** – despite quality help and support	
3.2	**Often very phonic** – sed, tayking, wos, becos	
3.3	**Unusual spelling** often with bizarre letter combinations	
3.4	**Letters out of sequence** and word reversal – was/saw, pin/nip, grils/girls, aply/play	
3.5	**Letter/number reversals** – b/d, p/q, often 4, 7, 9	
3.6	**Problems with blends** – cannot seem to put the sounds together	
3.7	**Problems with syllables**/ chunking words into sounds	
3.8	**Difficulty blending** sounds to spell words. Challenged by regular non/pseudo words - flimbat, vampeg.	
3.9	"Spells" during Literacy Hour but **rarely transfer skills** to other settings	
3.10	**Words spelt differently** within same paragraph/sentence	

3.1 Severe and persistent difficulties

- A classic dyslexic indicator, especially if others at the same level of ability and experience are making progress
- As long as spellings are not a "barrier to communication" – key exam phrase – then this does not need to be an issue
- Pay attention to the learner's emotional needs by not making an issue of the small words – they are important, but not at the expense of the feel-good factor
- Small words are often harder, because they lack a clear shape and pattern. Clapping and chunking are effective techniques, but – it is impossible to clap or chunk a one syllable word!
- If in doubt – ignore them until the learner is ready... Justify this approach through target marking but make sure parents understand what is happening and why
- Liaise with SENCO re: strategies that are working
- Focus on the use of ability appropriate language – more marks to be gained for this than will be lost through incorrect spelling of high frequency words
- If the above are not helping, mention to SENCO

3.2 Spellings often very phonic

Spellings like "gowing, layzy, tayking etc" indicate a failure to appreciate the difference between a word and a syllable. Work needs to be done on the "4 Rules of Spelling" with plenty of multi-sensory "Make and Break, Look, Cover, Write and Check" activities using the subject specific jargon words.

Give the learner a magnetic board, initially with all the letters needed to make the word and then add a few extra unnecessary letters as a challenge. This is very effective with jargon words.

3.3 Unusual or bizarre spelling

- Easier to deal with when the bizarre spelling is a consistent response. This indicates a likely confusion about some aspects of sound/syllable correspondence or blending rules and may be a case of substituting one response for another

- Much harder to address when the word is spelt in different ways at different times, indicating little idea of the structure of language. Ask for help/advice as this is way beyond what class/subject teachers should be expected to deal with – needs specialist intervention
- Use magnetic letters etc to "Make and Break – LCWC"
- May reflect visual problems if the learner cannot spot them during proof reading – try worksheets on coloured paper – also try producing lined paper on pastel shades
- Tactically ignore if the learner's current emotional needs dictate
- Ask the learner what is meant – if s/he does not know, refer to SENCO. Ask for help/advice as this is way beyond what teachers should be expected to deal with – specialist intervention/support needed

3.4/5   Letters/numbers out of sequence and/or number/word reversals

- Not a big deal unless it is a barrier to communication – tactically ignore wherever possible/appropriate
- Coloured paper, overlays etc may help
- Encourage learners to experiment with making reversed letters/numbers different
- In Maths, mark for content and process and be prepared to look for (and mark as correct) answers that work from right to left as well as from left to right

N.B. Writing capital letters in the middle of words can be a very intelligent response to not being sure of the orientation of the lower case letters. Writing "trouBle" gets round the problem nicely. In the first instance the learner deserves praise for developing an intelligent strategy to address the issue and then support to substitute the correct lower case letter.

- It is often more effective to associate the capital and the lower case pairings
- Do not labour the b/d difference - despite energetic teaching in the past it has never made sense to the learner and probably never will so try to address casually and with a variety of approaches.

- The learner may be able to come up with a strategy, given time and encouragement. Remember, "more means different"

3.6-8   Problems with blends and syllables

"Make and Break" is a useful strategy, as it has the inbuilt check of requiring all the letters given to be built into the word. Problems with polysyllabic jargon words also respond well to the following procedure:

- Print the word out several times, using font size 36 or bigger – choose the size to make the word as big as possible while remaining on one line
- Cut out the words, presenting the learner with words on strips of paper
- Ask the learner to "clap and tear" the word into syllables

Checkpoint

- Has each syllable got a vowel in it
- Does each syllable say what you want it to

Remember the 4 rules of spelling:

Single vowels say their **names** when they are:
1. On their own in a syllable (o/pen)
2. At the end of a syllable (e/mu)

Single vowels say their **sounds** when they are:
3. In the middle of a syllable (u/nit)
4. At the beginning of a syllable (ge/og/ra/phy)

This can become a useful "pair-share" activity, with a buddy checking and jumbling the syllables for more practice. When there is a sticking point with a particular letter combination, go back to individual letters and "Make and Break".

Using the remaining words, try asking the learner to clap the syllables again. Then to say the word out loud, "stretching it" to accentuate the syllable structure and marking the syllables with a forward slash. The final stage is to mark the syllables while reading it normally and then Look, Cover, Write, and Check.

Warning

Taught is not learnt – especially for dyslexic learners! This process works, but it may well need to be revisited with the same word over a period of time in order to achieve automaticity. However, time invested in getting the word right will pay off in the future. Exam markers do expect jargon words to be spelt correctly, or at least in a way which is not a barrier to communication. Each time a teacher invests time in Make and Break and syllabification, s/he is building skills for every teacher who will work with the learner in the future.

3.9 Spells in Literacy Hour or spelling tests but rarely transfers skills to other settings

A similar phenomenon may be observed in the learner who manages to achieve a respectable score in a spelling test but then fails to transfer the words correctly to free writing. This problem is due mainly to the use of a teaching style which is at odds with learner preferences, forcing them to work outside of their comfort zone. The skills taught within a literacy strategy need to be reinforced and over-learned through learner preferences if long term gains are to be secured. This may require a creative interpretation of the way the time is structured in order to secure the desired long term learning.

3.10 Words spelt differently within the same sentence/paragraph

Well-documented weaknesses with working memory make this simply something that dyslexic learners do – it can be a key indicator of specific problems, especially on "dyslexic days".

Putting pressure on the learner to pay more attention or to concentrate is counterproductive, can damage confidence and self-esteem and will probably make the situation worse.

However, acknowledging it as being "just one of those things" takes the pressure off and supports the learner to move on.

Try:

- Highlighting both spellings and ask the learner to choose
- Giving both spellings on a magnetic board and go for "Make and Break". Ask the learner to choose and then Look, Cover, Write, Check

In the early stages the learner may choose the wrong word, especially if it is a short word, with little pattern or shape. Try:

- Supporting the learner to identify any features of the correct word, e.g. "there" has "here" in it, so it is possible to link the notion of "here and there."
- Developing the concept of " serial probability" – the odds that certain letters usually come together

N.B. Refer to SENCO if difficulties persist despite quality intervention which is working with other learners who have apparently similar problems

4. SPEECH AND LANGUAGE

	Noted	Action
4.1 Problems **hearing the difference between sounds** – b/d, t/d, f/v/th,		
4.2 Persistently **inappropriate sounds in words** – pegals/pedals/ chimbley/chimney, shop bread/bread shop		
4.3 **Syllable omission/addition** – nucelar/nuclear, gong/going		
4.4 **Finding words/labels** – tends to use "thingy", "you know" etc		
4.5 **Problems remembering instructions** – easily overloaded		
4.6 Unexpected difficulty **understanding certain abstract concepts**		

4.1/2   Problems hearing the difference between sounds

- Confidence and self-esteem are paramount – this should never be allowed to become an issue for the learner

- This is a major challenge in a 1:1/small group situation, let alone in a mainstream setting. Best advice is to use Make and Break and also to present several possible "soundings" of the target word on a magnetic board – "bovver, bother" etc. As a rule of thumb, be prepared to celebrate the syllable structure and mark for that

N.B. Refer to SENCO if difficulties persist despite quality intervention which is working with other learners who have apparently similar problems

4.3 Syllable Omission/addition

Try:

- Giving the letters of the word, as spelt, on a magnetic board and going through Make and Break
- Ask" Does the word say what you want it to say? If not, how can you change it?"
- If the learner is happy with the way the word sounds we need to re-establish some basic principles at a later date
- There is nothing wrong with choosing to leave the issue for now, as long as it is returned to at an appropriate time – perhaps as part of a discrete intervention when the rest of the class are working independently

N.B. Refer to SENCO if difficulties persist despite quality intervention which is working with other learners who have apparently similar problems

4.4 Problems finding words and labels

Automatic word finding is a well documented issue for many dyslexic learners, especially when under pressure. The following strategies may help:

- Relax – both learner and teacher!
- Laugh about it with the learner – recognise that everybody has this problem, especially stressed teachers!
- Maintain eye contact, keep body language positive and resist the temptation to give the word, unless asked to do so - support as for learners who stammer

- Support in class to prevent other learners from reinforcing feelings of inadequacy by shouting out the word

4.5 Unexpected difficulties remembering instructions

Another classic sign of a specific learning difference, especially if recall is fine when instructions are given in different ways or when the learner is following her/his own process or procedure.

Sound advice is to use a routine for calling the class to order –perhaps by the teacher always standing in the same place, use the same words, same gestures, and have the same expectations each time. I always stand at the front of the class and in the middle of the board, when I call for attention. If I am not "on the spot" when I want attention, I will move before I speak. This seems to help learners to focus – they know where I will be, look up and there I am. If they have to look around to find me they easily get distracted and I have lost them before I start. Then:

- Think before speaking – mentally chunk into positive, "do-able" bite sized chunks
- Say what you want – not what you don't want
- Say what you mean and mean what you say – if it is essential that everyone stops writing, puts pens down and looks up, then everyone must do it. The lesson must not progress until that series of instructions has been followed by all learners
- Use a simple rule of thumb:
  - If it is important enough to stop everyone working, then everyone must do what is asked (e.g. pens down, fold your arms)
  - Do not continue until everyone has followed the instruction
  - If everyone does not have to do it, why ask everyone to do it in the first place?

- Responses to individuals will vary according to need. I usually insist on eye contact from all learners when I am giving instructions, though I am aware that, for some, this is a real challenge. In that case I am prepared to accept a raise of the head to indicate that I have been heard – learners with autism appreciate this concession, as do most adolescents.

The important principle is to acknowledge differences in preference and respond in a flexible way which achieves attention without confrontation

- Learners who are choosing not to focus respond well to a warning that, at the end of the instruction sequence, I will ask people to tell their partners what is to be done or select people to repeat what I said

- Dyslexic learners may also suffer from speech and language problems – if problems persist, despite the use of good practice which is working for others, refer to your SENCO

4.6 Difficulty understanding certain abstract concepts

- This may be a "readiness" issue relating to the fact that the development of understanding is a stage by stage process; the attainment of one stage depends on the full integration of the one before. In consequence a learner who is not "ready" will find it difficult to understand certain concepts. This issue is addressed, in part, by the notion of the spiral curriculum and there is a responsibility on us all to ensure that concepts are re-visited

- Another likely cause is that the concept has been presented in a way "uncomfortable" for the learner. That is to say outside of the comfortable range of learning styles and preferences. The key here is to present the concept so that it is accessible through a range of learning styles and to actively encourage a variety of possible responses

- Peer tutoring opportunities can help to develop and firm up concepts. It may seem threatening to require a confused learner to explain a concept to another but it can work well. The emotional climate of the classroom holds the key – if collaborative learning is well established and it is safe to make mistakes then learners will have the confidence to push the boundaries of their knowledge and skill to teach a friend

5. WRITING

	Noted	Action
5.1 Quantity of writing - rarely matches range of ideas expressed orally		
5.2 Quality of writing – rarely matches quality of ideas expressed orally		
5.3 Quality of vocabulary – often poor in comparison to ideas expressed orally		
5.4 Getting started – needs support to begin		
5.5 Lacks confidence in writing activities – easily put off/intimidated by task		
5.6 Spelling deteriorates when in the flow of writing		
5.7 Organisation of ideas – difficulties with paragraphing		
5.8 Sequencing of ideas – difficulties with the order of ideas/information		
5.9 Punctuation - non-existent or random		

5.1/2 Quantity and quality of writing rarely matches ideas

Getting it down on paper can be difficult for dyslexic learners, and getting started is often the real challenge - the response of the teacher will determine whether this issue is a learning difference or becomes a learning difficulty. If the following strategies work, then the issue is possibly due to a specific learning difference – in this case the learner cannot currently produce ability appropriate writing in the way demanded, but can produce excellent evidence of thinking or understanding in other forms. Try:

- Inviting the learner to choose a preferred way to present or plan the activity
- Drawing a mind map for, or with, the learner
- Asking for a brainstorm of everything the learner wants to write – then re-process using colour, strips of paper, post-its etc
- Starting with a storyboard
- Developing a flow chart
- Pair/share tasks – learners tell each other what they intend to write
- Giving sentence or paragraph starters – this is really effective

- Giving paragraph starters but challenge learners to modify to suit their needs
- Using a framework
- Asking another adult or a peer to scribe for part/all of the activity
- Using speech/write technology

Asking the learner to present the information as a broadcast/news item on web cam or video

5.3 Poor written expression compared to oral contribution

Dyslexic learners need support to strike a balance between fluent expression and a need for accurate spelling. Uninspiring written language may reflect an undue preoccupation with accuracy at the expense of style. Although understandable, it will be penalized in exam situations. Try:

- Encouraging learners to "go for it" and use "classy words" at all times
- Supporting them by target marking and "tactically ignoring" certain aspects
- Encouraging learners to ask for words and tell them without any "teaching"
- Use adjective/noun grids to support writing in all subjects – learners list the nouns they intend to use in the right hand column.
- The task then is to add two appropriate adjectives to each noun, and then select the most effective combination for the task in hand (This approach also works well for verbs and adverbs)

Adjectives	Noun

5.4/5 Problems getting started/ lacking confidence

See 5.1/2 above

5.6 Spelling deteriorates when in the flow of writing

Dyslexic learners need to work very much harder than their peers to develop and maintain their secretarial skills – they may need to work up to five times harder! In consequence there may not be much headroom left to facilitate writing as well, so something has to go.

My preference is to ask for quality of expression and information processing, if necessary at the expense of spelling, and my pupils know of this preference. In consequence the deterioration of spelling is not usually an issue in my classroom. I reinforce this principle with carefully considered target marking.

Spelling will improve when learners have a clear idea of the order of information to be presented and when they are working from a plan which matches their learning preferences.

5.7/8 Organising and/or sequencing ideas – difficulties with paragraphs

- Inviting the learner to choose a preferred way to present or plan the activity
- Drawing a mind map for, or with, the learner
- Asking for a brainstorm of everything the learner wants to write – then re-process using colour, strips of paper, post-its etc
- Starting with a storyboard
- Developing a flow chart
- Pair/share tasks – learners tell each other what they intend to write
- Giving sentence or paragraph starters – this is really effective
- Giving paragraph starters but challenge learners to modify to suit their needs
- Using a framework
- Asking another adult or a peer to scribe for part/all of the activity
- Using speech/write technology

Try using colour – either from a mind map or by colour coding information to organize information processing.

5.9 Punctuation

Dyslexic learners often find it difficult to do more than one thing at a time when in the flow of writing. In consequence the secretarial skill of punctuation may often be forgotten. If the learner is actually writing in sentences but not punctuating try:

- Asking him/her to read it to you and "punctuate the pauses"
- Finding a capital letter, put a full stop in after 3 sentences and ask the learner to put in two more full stops – asking for a target number of full stops within a clearly defined number of lines is effective
- Delineating a few lines of prose, with a capital letter and a full stop and asking for the necessary number of full stops etc to be added

6. PRESENTATION

	Noted	Action
6.1 Slow handwriting - often painfully slow		
6.2 Tires easily/quickly		
6.3 Inefficient grip – may shake hand, massage fingers, etc		
6.4 Poorly formed/shaped letters despite adequate practice		
6.5 Reversals - b/d, p/q, was/saw, etc		
6.6 Inappropriate capital letters - often in the middle of words		
6.7 Poor page layout – may write down the middle of the page or over to the right		
6.8 No preferred hand – not sure which hand to use to write		
6.9 Laterality– not sure in which direction to write		

To be judged only against an individual's best efforts rather than against any external standard. The first pages of an exercise book are often a reflection of "best" work so a fair benchmark is to compare current presentation with these pages.

6.1/2 Slow handwriting/tires easily

- This can be due, in part, to dyspraxia. Also it may be "learned helplessness" in response to pressure. The logic goes, "If I write slowly, I won't have to do as much and perhaps someone will do it for me"

Try:

- Comparing handwriting speed when the learner is keen and has chosen to write – if speed does increase then a lack of speed may be a choice in response to certain tasks
- Stating a minimum number of lines or sentences to be completed – be fair and reasonable, but firm
- Offering a deal to chunk the task – "You write the first 5 lines and you can dictate the rest to me" or "I'll get you started and you write me ….. more lines"
- Accepting work in different forms

6.3   Inefficient Grip

- Regardless of the age of the learner, trying to change a pen or pencil grip is seeking to change the habits of a lifetime
- There are various grips that can be slipped over a pen or pencil and these can work well.   A large lump of blue tack or plasticine on the pen can also encourage the hand to open up.   However it is important to be aware that these strategies may also make the learner feel stigmatized
- Older learners respond well to being challenged to fine tune their grip for comfort, bearing in mind that the most comfortable is often no change whatsoever!
- Inviting learners to look at the grips used by others can be a gentle way of making a point, especially if different grips are linked to writing speed and writer comfort i.e. "Paul can write at 20 words/minute with his grip and Jane can write at 18 words/minute using hers and they can both write for a long time. You are writing at 7 words a minute and your hand hurts after a couple of minutes. What conclusions can you draw from this?"

6.4 Poorly formed/shaped letters

- Teachers may need to be prepared to lose the battle for well shaped letters in order to win the war of communication through writing

- Various NC criteria seem to place pressure on learners and teachers alike to develop a cursive, joined up script, often at the expense of communication when "joined up" for some means illegible

- I would argue that the only point of writing is to communicate and there is no long term virtue in developing a "good hand", especially as text, e-mail etc become the norm – as they are already. If this is accepted it becomes apparent that writing which is printed and legible is automatically better that writing which is joined up and illegible

- Most teachers will know learners who actually write much faster and communicate more effectively by printing

- There is an understandable concern about "losing marks" in SATs etc. However I have watched learners cease to communicate through the adoption of a joined up style and lose even more marks because their work is illegible. If this argument makes sense, schools may need to consider adding a note in an appropriate policy document to make clear why all learners are encouraged to develop a style of writing which enables them to communicate effectively

- Specially prepared paper may help. Try creating lined paper with a middle line to determine the height of lower case letters. This paper is particularly effective with two modifications:

  1. Shade the lower half of the line – this seems to make it easier for learners to "see" the need for height differentials between letters

  2. Print on pastel paper – this cuts down the visual processing problems associated with black print on a white background

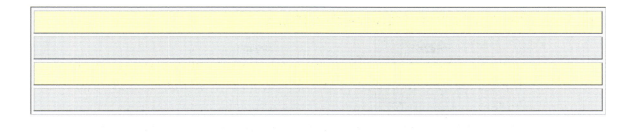

the octopus is scary.

6.5/6   Reversals and inappropriate capitals

Letter reversals are going to happen throughout a dyslexic learner's life and really are no big deal – certainly I would not be worrying too much about them in a mainstream lesson as I am more concerned with concept development and the effective processing of information. It follows, then, that the reversal of letter strings within words (siad, thier etc) will probably happen throughout life as well, especially under pressure, and should be an equally low priority issue providing that the spelling is not a barrier to communication. Choosing to identify reversals as part of a target marking strategy may be appropriate, especially if it leads to coordinated action to improve – just crossing out/correcting reversals during a "death by deep marking" exercise is pointless, unhelpful and a waste of time for both teacher and learner.

Putting capital letters in the middle of words is an intelligent response from learners who know they have a reversal problem with lower case letters but can tell them apart as capitals – writing "BeD" solves the problem very quickly and effectively. It is worth investing time across the curriculum to support learners to deal with this issue but, once again, probably not at the expense of efficient and effective communication. It is worth remembering that there are dyslexic learners at university who still rely on this strategy. Also there are envious non dyslexic young people who have no problems with reversals etc and who would like to go to university but could not get the grades!

6.7 Poor page layout

Dyslexic and Dyspraxic learners may share a lack of awareness of the importance of the left hand margin as the place to start writing. These learners may also be seriously challenged by being required to write in boxes and to fill in gaps as part of a cloze exercise. In consequence they may find it difficult to show what they know in multi-choice type assessments.

Drawing bold margins on both sides of a page seems to help, as does forgetting about paragraphs for a while. Sometimes starting in from the margin for the paragraph causes the next line to start even further in, and so on. Persistent reminders to write down the left hand margin and to get close to the right hand margin seem to help, providing the main preoccupation is with the learner's self esteem – the effective communication of ideas down the right hand side of a page is arguably better than boring rubbish laid out "properly". This does seem to be another "readiness" issue for many learners and one which may require specialist intervention so a referral to the SENCO may be indicated. In the meantime "accentuate the positive", use the language of success wherever possible.

6.8/9 No preferred hand and/or not sure in which direction to write

The mainstream teacher's response to these issues needs to be part of a coordinated approach involving the SENCO. As the learner grows older these issues become more and more atypical and will require increasingly urgent intervention. It becomes the class/subject teacher's responsibility to ensure that any discrete intervention strategies are supported and reinforced across all subjects and at all times.

Dyslexic learners will, quite commonly, write from left to right for the first line, then right to left for the next and so on. Often just pointing this out is enough to stop it. Placing a dot at the left hand side of each line, together with the instruction "Start at the dot" can also help. What is essential is that all teachers have the same expectations and follow the same strategies as stipulated by the SENCO. It is also important that all demands pay due attention to the learner's self esteem.

7. MATHEMATICS

	Noted	Action
7.1 **Confusion** with place value		
7.2 Choosing the **correct process**		
7.3 **Remembering** mathematical symbols		
7.4 **Reversals** – of individual numbers and strings of numbers		
7.5 **Learning tables**, number bonds, anything in a sequence		
7.6 Problems with **mental maths**		
7.7 **Reading** the question		
7.8 Telling the **time**		

7.1/2 Confusion with place value and choosing the correct process

- Use graph paper to support accurate setting out of sums in all subjects
- Keep it kinaesthetic – hands on place value activities will support development of the concept
- Keep it real and go for "ball park figures" – rounding up and rounding down to get a "guesstimate" that fits. Then go back and look at place values and process
- Ensure new information links with previous knowledge

7.3 Remembering mathematical symbols

- Use the language of maths at every opportunity to link words and symbols
- Precision teaching is effective – short quizzes to over-learn the relationship between symbol and process
- Ensure new information links with previous knowledge – essential to work from inside out
- Be prepared to go back to re-learn/re-emphasise early concepts and skills

- Framework the maths to ensure that the acquisition of important numerical concepts in, say, History or Science do not founder on the mechanics of the sums

7.4 Reversals

- Be prepared for reversals – likely to be a constant issue for dyslexic learners
- Mark for process – insist working is shown to enable the teacher to back track. Learner resistance to showing the working can be countered by unpacking the marking process and demonstrating:

    1. How many marks are available for a well-worked answer which is wrong
    2. How reversed number strings can be right if the working gives a clue

7.5 Learning tables

- Likely to be a nightmare for many dyslexic learners – the learning process targets many typical areas of weakness, so be gentle!
- Invest time in number bonds and the relationship between numbers – precision teaching gives an effective return for the time invested
- Look for "free gifts" – 3x6 gives the learner 6x3

7.6 Mental maths

- Likely to be a nightmare for many dyslexic learners – mental maths targets many typical areas of weakness, so be aware, take the pressure off and be gentle!
- Also likely to be very stressful unless tricks of the trade, like the right to pass, are in place
- Consider working a small group separately with another adult or a peer to lead the activity
- Wherever possible, use pair/share activities
- Give take up time
- Give hands on materials to support thinking

7.7 Reading the question

- Teach, reinforce and over-learn the language – and be prepared to do it again and again. "Taught is learnt" is not a mantra for a Dyslexia Friendly school
- Reinforce key words and phrases with flash cards, precision teaching etc
- Explain to partner - pair/share activities work well
- Transform the question into a mind map or story board – answering the "who, what, why, where, when, how" questions will support comprehension
- Go for guesstimates – require learners to articulate and justify their ball park figure and reduce stress by asking for an answer with a wide "plus or minus" range

7.8 Telling the time

- Go digital – for simplicity and expediency
- Practice the language – peer tutoring and precision teaching
- Give take up time
- Likely to be a "readiness" issue so be prepared to marginalise the importance until the learner is clearly ready

Chapter 14

SCHOOL IMPROVEMENT THROUGH DYSLEXIA FRIENDLY BEST PRACTICE

Before embarking upon what could be perceived as just another initiative it is essential to be able to answer the "WIIFME" (What's In It For Me) question.   The purpose of this chapter is to support Senior Managers and SENCOs to justify taking the school down a Dyslexia Friendly route and to make a case for using Dyslexia Friendly fine tuning as the unifying and coordinating medium for some major imperatives in schools today, specifically:

- Every Child Matters
- Inspectorate Key Questions
- School Self Evaluation (SEF)

The chart "Measuring the Journey" shows how these elements can be combined to create a self evaluation strategy in which data is collected once but used in a variety of ways. The key questions asked by the Inspectorate encourage schools to target groups of pupils as part of a self assessment strategy. Making dyslexic pupils the focus of such scrutiny could be seen as a logical first step in examining the effectiveness of a school's inclusivity and effectiveness. The chart also works well as the first part of a two stage training exercise, the second of which will be presented at the end of the chapter. Teams address the issues and brainstorm available evidence to write on to the chart. At the end of the exercise it is clear at a glance which areas are strong and which are in need of attention.

Measuring the Journey - 1

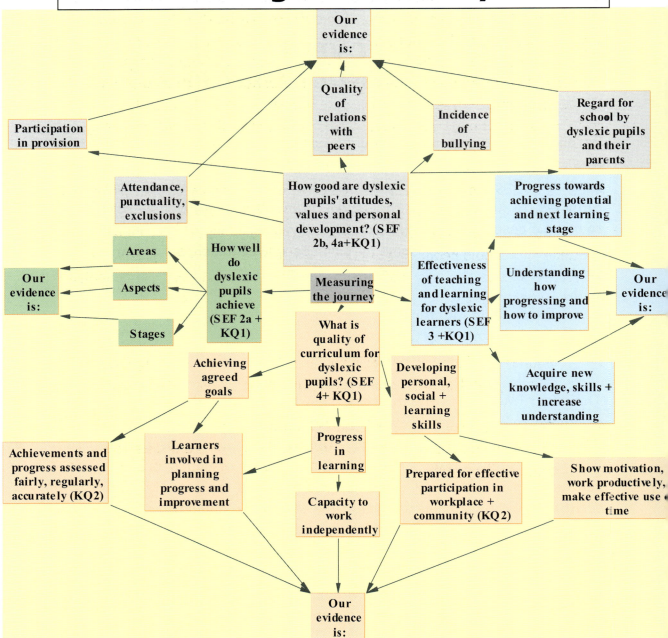

Long experience of promoting whole school change shows the importance of ensuring that current or future directions are built in to the School Improvement Plan. This document plots the direction of initiatives over a number of years and is an important vehicle for managing change. The exercise described above can feed into the school improvement plan to reflect new imperatives which have been arrived at consensually – something which may not always happen when new directions are being planned.

Reports by Inspectors give a very clear steer regarding central priorities for schools based on many hundreds of inspections. An analysis of Section 5 reports, as set out in the chart below, sends a very clear message to schools regarding current and future priorities, priorities which are also at the heart of a Dyslexia Friendly initiative. This analysis has the potential to:

1. Support colleagues to begin to make their case for using Dyslexia Friendly best practice as a main thrust for school improvement

2. Show how a focus on Dyslexia Friendly issues for learning and teaching has the potential to address many of the issues raised in Section 5 reports

Section 5 Reports

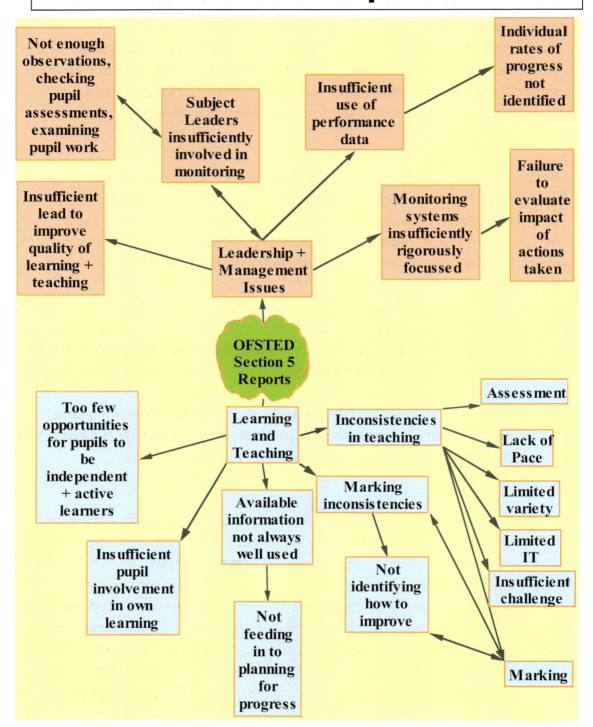

Leadership and Management

Inspectors use the school self assessment data to ask Leaders and Managers a range of questions about a range of issues. They listen carefully to the answers and then ask the key question, "How do you know – where/what is your evidence?" The quality of monitoring and evaluation is currently seen as an issue for the Inspectorate, specifically with regard to the focus/rigor of monitoring systems, the involvement of team/subject leaders in the process and the use of performance data to guide learning and teaching. Discussions with teachers around the UK suggest these issues to be common concerns, with many schools planning to address them at some stage but not quite sure how best to move forward.

One expectation is that schools look at the outcomes of different groups within their community to assess where pupils are in relation to others within their group and also with regard to those in other groups. At first sight this can be a daunting task – where to start is the problem. However strategies to meet the needs of Dyslexic pupils have already been put forward as offering whole class/whole school based benefits across a range of learning needs. Therefore it makes sense to break the task down into bite sized chunks and make dyslexic pupils the "target group" for a monitoring initiative by team and subject leaders with a particular focus on improving the quality of learning and teaching by:

- Getting into classrooms to check pupil assessments and work
- Sharing performance data with class/subject teachers to identify and track the rates of progress of dyslexic learners
- Evaluate the impact of Dyslexia Friendly fine tuning

A particular thrust could be to recognize that the Inspectorate is not just interested in where pupils have arrived – the point of departure and the quality of the journey are equally important. Therefore there is a real opportunity to work with colleagues to find creative ways of measuring the distance travelled by Dyslexic learners and coordinate a whole school response to the information gathered. The training and learning that takes place during this exercise with a small and clearly defined group can then be transferred to a more comprehensive roll out in the certain knowledge that issues identified and resolved on behalf of this target group will almost invariably enhance the learning of all in the school.

Learning and Teaching

As with Leadership and Management, the Learning and Teaching issues also seem to be common to a majority of schools across the UK and beyond. Once again, placing the focus on a clearly definable group of dyslexic learners makes the task instantly more manageable but with obvious opportunities for a more inclusive roll out once basic principles and strategies are in place.

Once Team and Subject Leaders take a lead in requiring performance data to inform and direct learning and teaching of dyslexic learners, it is a small step for class and subject teachers to ensure that this data feeds into planning for progress. As will be shown later, the emphasis on listening to the pupil voice, which is a key element of Every Child Matters, enables teachers to individualise learning very effectively and also to identify generic elements by cross referencing individual preferences. Given the opportunity to voice an opinion, most pupils seem to value involvement in their own learning and the opportunity to be active and independent. Obviously these approaches will suit the eclectic, often kinesthetic preferences of dyslexic learners, but there are likely to be few learners in any classroom anywhere who do not prefer to be actively engaged in their learning. It was a girl in a Liverpool Primary School who voiced her frustration at not being given time to reflect on learning. Her perception was that as soon as something had been taught, the class moved on to something else, whereas her preference was to come back to it during the next lesson to reflect and consolidate what had gone before. The policy of listening to the voice of the pupil has already led to changes in learning and teaching in the school.

> # Two out of every three children need a good listening to!

Leaders and managers also have the opportunity to offer a positive steer with regard to the sorts of reasonable adjustments that are part of a school's commitment to Quality First teaching. One of the easiest ways to measure a pupil's journey is to offer them choice in the way in which

212

evidence of learning is presented. Saying "You choose" immediately engages learners, offering opportunities for independence and involvement.

Inconsistencies in teaching are a concern for many Head Teachers and, as a basic principle, all learners are entitled to a basic level of awareness and facilitation of their intellectual, social and emotional needs – it must not be a lottery which teacher a child gets! The monitoring role of Team and Subject leaders defined by the Inspectorate requires inconsistencies to be identified where they occur, which is in the classroom, and then addressed by performance management. As before, focusing on dyslexic learners in the first instance defines a manageable cohort from which best practice can spiral outward and upward.

To turn the discussion on its head and hark back to the "School that I'd like" section earlier in the book, imagine the quality of learning for dyslexic learners when all available information is used to inform and direct planning for progress. The improvement in learning which accrues when pupils are independent and active will have been closely monitored and fine tuned to ensure a consistency of teaching, a house style which defines and stipulates the reasonable adjustments that learners can expect; in other words their basic entitlement to Quality First teaching is transparent and understood by all. The concept of house style is possibly the key – the Foundation Stage Profile in England already stresses the importance of a seamless transition between stages, pointing out how learning suffers for protracted periods of time if the gap between stages is too great. Therefore a house style at Key Stage 2 which embraces and harnesses the best of Key Stage 1 can only serve to help and support sensitive and/or vulnerable learners, with the same principle applying between Key Stages 2 and 3. A house style which offers a variety of assessment techniques and "evidence opportunities" which are based on pupil preference, designed to measure the learning journey with an appropriate balance of challenge and supported by assistive technology where appropriate will empower dyslexic learners to be the best they can be. Let us forget Dyslexia Friendly for a minute – this sounds very much like assessment for learning. In fact it sounds like best practice across the typical range of learning needs in any school anywhere!

A house style which offers a variety of assessment techniques and "evidence opportunities" which are:

- based on pupil preference
- designed to measure the learning journey with an appropriate balance of challenge
- supported by assistive technology where appropriate

will empower dyslexic learners to be the best they can be

The purpose of this section was to demonstrate how issues for management, learning and teaching identified in OFSTED/ESTYN Section 5 reports may be tackled through a small scale Dyslexia Friendly imitative. Once Leaders and Managers have evaluated the positive impact of actions taken on behalf of dyslexic learners it is but a small step to fine tune learning and teaching across the range of need and to empower all learners to experience the joy and beauty of success.

The next section puts Dyslexia Friendly firmly into the context of Every Child Matters and demonstrates how pursuing one agenda cannot help but define and promote the other.

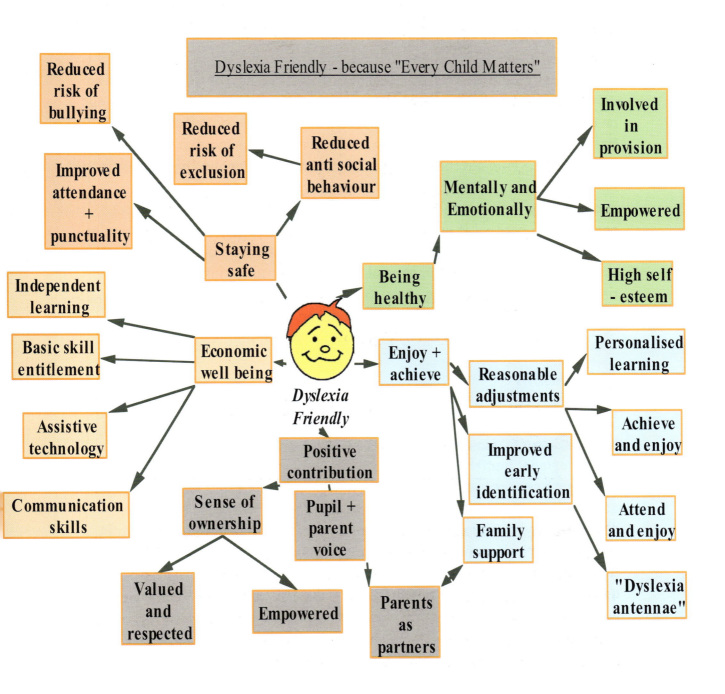

Dyslexia Friendly - because "Every Child Matters"

Reduced risk of bullying

Improved attendance + punctuality

Reduced risk of exclusion

Reduced anti social behaviour

Staying safe

Mentally and Emotionally

Involved in provision

Empowered

High self - esteem

Being healthy

Independent learning

Basic skill entitlement

Economic well being

Assistive technology

Communication skills

Dyslexia Friendly

Enjoy + achieve

Reasonable adjustments

Personalised learning

Achieve and enjoy

Improved early identification

Attend and enjoy

Positive contribution

Pupil + parent voice

Sense of ownership

Family support

"Dyslexia antennae"

Valued and respected

Empowered

Parents as partners

There is an obvious imperative to develop whole school responses to Every Child Matters and some schools are already basing their Improvement Plans on the 5 outcomes. As ever, the question will always be "How do you know it is working/making a difference?" and, as ever, it makes sense to begin the monitoring process with a clearly defined target group. The chart above shows how a Dyslexia Friendly thrust can be used to obtain evidence of success.

Staying safe:

The safest place for dyslexic learners to be during the school day is in school. However they often vote with their feet by contriving absences or arriving late if they feel vulnerable. Therefore one outcome of becoming more Dyslexia Friendly is likely to be improved attendance and punctuality. This outcome is already documented among Dyslexia Friendly schools, as are reduced numbers of exclusions. As learners are successfully included in the learning process and empowered to exercise appropriate control it would also be reasonable to expect a reduction in anti social behaviour. Finally schools which celebrate diversity and actively promote social, emotional and intellectual inclusion are likely to be places in which bullying is much less likely to happen. These outcomes are easy to identify on a "before and after" basis and also link conveniently with data required for self evaluation. (SEF)

Being healthy

Sadly the notion of healthy schools seems to be associated mainly with physical issues. However I intend to focus this outcome on the mental and emotional health and well being which comes from high self esteem, a culture of respect and empowerment through success. Many schools are actively engaged in measuring and developing self esteem through a commitment to Social and Emotional Aspects of Learning (SEAL) and other initiatives and it makes sense to focus on a target group like dyslexic learners in order to make evaluation manageable. The disparity between ability and performance can make this group particularly vulnerable so measures which work for them will probably work for all.

Empowerment through reasonable adjustments and differentiation by outcome based on learning styles and preferences also contributes to social and emotional health. Success indicators will probably be shared with the Staying Safe strand plus that essential element, pupil and parental confidence. This comes from learners and parents being engaged and involved in decisions about provision and empowered to contribute to final outcomes. Schools which are actively listening to the voices of pupils and parents report benefits in many areas and collect evidence in a variety of ways including increased attendance at Parent and Child evenings, reduction in phone calls etc and often set out to establish a "good news" file of letters, phone call transcripts and emails from

216

parents which acknowledge when things are going well. I saw this done very effectively in a school in Warwickshire which linked parental communication logs with samples of the child's work and, over time, it was possible to track how parental confidence, as evidenced by letters etc, increased with the quality of the child's work. This evidence was a fascinating record and most compelling.

Enjoy and achieve

This strand is about the "reasonable adjustments" that all teachers can make of behalf of dyslexic learners as part of a commitment to Quality First teaching.   In a Dyslexia Friendly school these adjustments are based on awareness of the needs of dyslexic learners, but do not require a label before they can be made. So Dyslexia Friendly schools are not requiring teachers to label children as being dyslexic, but rather enabling them to develop their "dyslexia antennae" in order to:

1. Identify children who would benefit from a Dyslexia Friendly approach
2. Make appropriate reasonable adjustments needed to take a learner forward.
3. Monitor in order to assess viability of any fine tuning – is it working?

Forget looking for labels. Instead ask class/subject teachers to:

- Identify children who would benefit from a Dyslexia Friendly approach

- Make appropriate reasonable adjustments needed to take a learner forward

- Monitor in order to assess viability of any fine tuning – is it working?

Compelling evidence will centre around the ability and willingness of teachers to adopt broader approaches to evidence of achievement for those learners who cannot currently deliver via standard outcomes. Consider a learner who is finding it very difficult to provide evidence of learning in written form. There can be little logic in wasting the child's time to develop cursive script when evidence of the journey towards ability appropriate achievement can be generated via assistive technology, web cam, Dictaphone or scribe. I know that cursive script is an element of SATs but, in the world that operates at Key Stage 4 and beyond, the issue is about what is communicated, not how well letters are formed. Also bear in mind that in further and higher education, coursework is unlikely to be accepted if handwritten – the expectation is that it will be word processed. Therefore keyboard skills are likely to be much more important than a "fair hand" in terms of future life chances.

When these adjustments do not work, as will happen with some children, Dyslexia ceases to become a specific learning difference and becomes a difficulty which requires specialist intervention. The chart below shows effective strategies identified by the Inspectorate –they all look pretty Dyslexia Friendly to me and serve to emphasise just how much quality first good practice is taking place in classrooms all over the UK. It also indicates how little fine tuning is required in order to be even more effective, initially for Dyslexic learners and then across the range of learning needs.

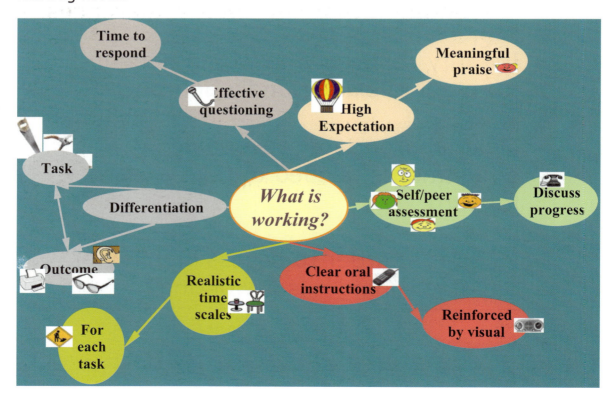

Listening to the voice of the pupil which is informed by a metacognitive appreciation of learning styles and preferences will make an important contribution to a learner's enjoyment and achievement. Learning which is personalised for success is a unifying factor across Dyslexia Friendly and ECM and will result in a range of success indicators including improved attendance/punctuality figures and any number of creative measures schools can dream up to provide evidence pupil journeys from where they were to where they are now. Parents also find the evidence fascinating and value this form of concrete evidence of success.

In other words we should trust our Pupils to:

- **Interpret a task** according to their learning preferences (SEF5b+ Personalised Learning + Excellence and Enjoyment + Removing Barriers + DFS)

- **Choose appropriate methods** of presentation that suit their preferences (SEF4 + Personalised Learning + Removing Barriers + DFS)

- **Provide evidence** in appropriate and acceptable ways (SEF3 + Excellence and Enjoyment + Removing Barriers + DFS)

Making a positive contribution

The sense of ownership that is a basic requirement of good mental and emotional health is also part of feeling able to make a positive contribution. The key here is to empower and respond to the voice of the pupil and the voice of the parent, especially for learners who do not have IEPs. Pupils who know how they learn best and are aware of strategies that work for them can make informed choices. Parents live with their dyslexic children and often have very clear ideas about what is effective and what is not. Schools which are encouraging the voices of pupils and parents are reaping all manner of rewards as they come to recognise the importance of being a "listening school".

Economic well-being

Although this can seem a long way off for younger children, it can never be too early to begin to develop skills. Dyslexia Friendly schools encourage the development of learning situations which enable pupils to work independently to solve problems – this is becoming particularly evident in schools which adopt the "I can" ethos. Assistive technology is improving all the time and, once exam boards respond to the march of progress, speech write technology will empower many dyslexic learners to be the best they can be in exam situations. Schools are also working incredibly hard to honour every child's entitlement to a basic level of literacy and numeracy skill together with the development of those vital communication skills which are the foundation of being "employable".

Pulling the threads together

When I talk to teachers during my presentations I am sometimes struck by a perceived sense of helplessness as they struggle to respond to wave after wave of initiatives, strategies and requests for data across a whole range of apparently unconnected areas. The Dyslexia Friendly initiative offers schools a unifying medium through which to establish monitoring and evaluation strategies for a clearly defined and manageable cohort before going "whole school" in the certain knowledge that best practice for dyslexic learners is probably best practice for all. This is perhaps best illustrated by using a fine tuned version of the "Measuring the Journey" chart (page 207).

However instead of asking for evidence of current practice, the focus is now on how to fine tune current practice in order to generate a 5% improvement in each area. This forms the second part of the training activity described at the beginning of the chapter as teachers are challenged to reflect on a series of manageable small steps in order to be even more effective.

Measuring the Journey - 2

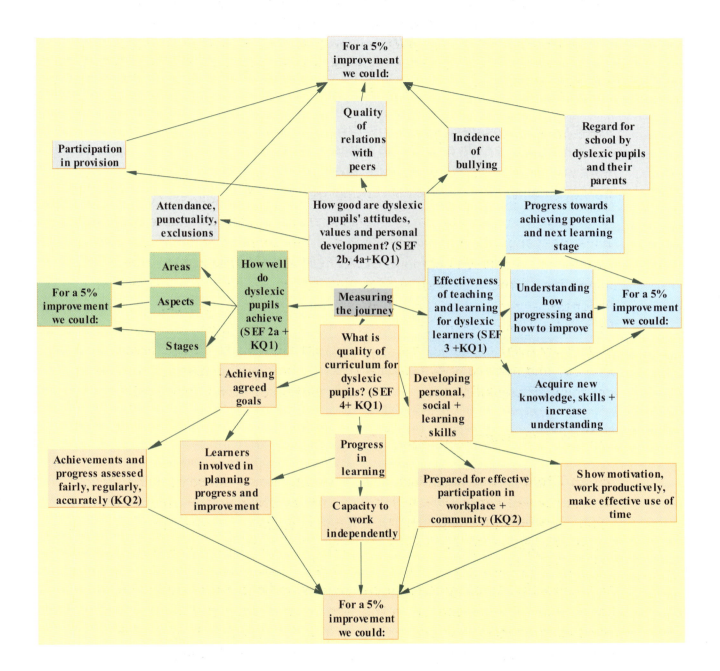

This is a powerful activity, but teachers often need to be supported to go for small steps rather than the big fix. My view is that most teachers are Dyslexia Friendly to varying degrees for much of their time – the challenge, as identified in the OFSTED/ESTYN Section 5 reports, is to reduce inconsistencies in teaching and to raise the quality of each learner's basic entitlement to Quality First teaching supported by a repertoire of reasonable adjustments. Teachers also have very high standards and they can find it difficult to appreciate how minimal fine tuning can make a significant difference. Often it is a language issue – I have been much more effective since I stopped saying "What is the answer?" which limits pupils to responses which are basically right or wrong and started asking "What answers could there be?" in order to encourage creative responses and risk taking.

It may only be a drop in the ocean, but Mother Teresa pointed out how important it is to put the drop in the right ocean. Fine tuning to generate a 5% improvement in any of the areas identified in the chart will almost invariably have a knock on effect, not only in other areas, but also for other children outside the current target group.

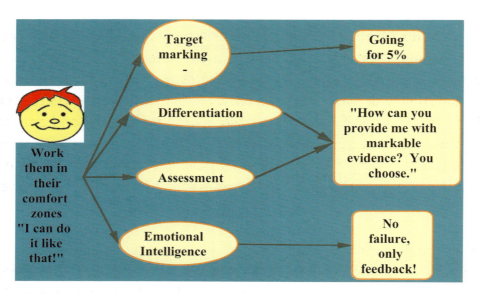

Things to do on Monday

Summary

How to use a Dyslexia Friendly initiative to achieve a coherent response to:

- Every Child Matters
- Inspectorate Key Questions
- Self Evaluation

Chapter 15

THE DYSLEXIA FRIENDLY CLASSROOM IN THE DYSLEXIA FRIENDLY SCHOOL

From Classroom to School

There will be Dyslexia Friendly classrooms in schools throughout the UK and beyond. Also there is an ever increasing number of Dyslexia Friendly schools which are being supported and accredited through innovative schemes organised by creative and forward thinking Children's Services. The British Dyslexia Association is liaising with a number of these to coordinate and build on this existing good practice and has established a national Quality Mark.

To achieve this Quality Mark, Children's Services submit themselves for scrutiny against stringent criteria and, once successful, are able to accredit their own Dyslexia Friendly Schools with an award which carries a national standard. An important feature of the accreditation process is for Services to establish rigorous systems for monitoring and evaluating their schools with regard to the successful identification and teaching of dyslexic pupils. Many Services already have effective strategies in place and there are clear links with initiatives such as the Basic Skills Kitemark.

However the prime focus continues to be on Dyslexic learners in mainstream classrooms and the quality of inclusive support to enable them to be the best they can be. The initial challenge is to translate discrete classroom based good practice into whole school good practice so that, as dyslexic learners move through the school and through the timetable, they can rely on an informed and empathic response from all contact teachers at all times in all lessons. Having achieved this, the next challenge is to enshrine good practice in policy and to use policy to drive and extend good practice even further.

Starting with Inclusion

The problem with traditional SEN approaches is that a learner has to fail, often for an unacceptably long time, in order to qualify for help. Funding is currently linked to labels and the only way to get one is often to jump through "assessment hoops" while going steadily backwards in terms of skill acquisition and, all too often, in terms of confidence and self esteem.

One solution is to put inclusion at the heart of everything a school does and to reflect this by placing inclusion at the centre of the school's policy web so that it guides and informs everything. It also serves to keep the learner as the focal point of policy and practice.

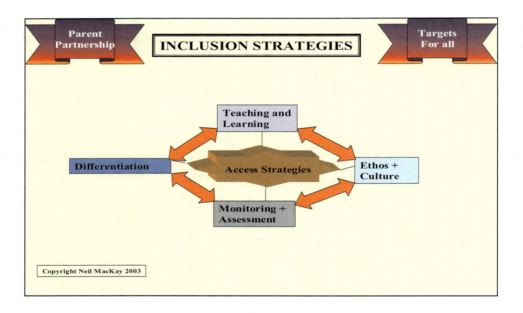

This simplified policy web shows how inclusion can begin to inform four key policies for a school. It is then possible to put some meat onto the bones of the skeleton in order to translate policy into classroom based good practice.

The Policy Web

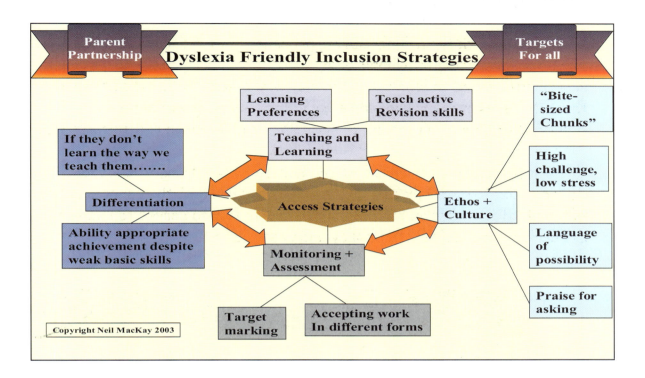

Ethos and culture make an appropriate starting point, because these elements are at the heart of a Dyslexia Friendly school. Most teachers (and Inspectors) will know of schools with the most wonderful paper policies, colour coordinated, beautifully bound and kept in the Head's office where they are insulated from all harm and all influence. Unfortunately these policies often have little bearing on what happens in the classroom and especially on the way vulnerable learners are treated. However teachers in a Dyslexia Friendly school will communicate their total conviction that progress will be made, through language, selection of learning tasks and interaction with pupils.

The ethos and culture of the school becomes translated into action through the teaching and learning policy. This policy is likely to be based around learning styles and preferences to achieve a mind friendly learning environment for all pupils. Learners will also be taught how to learn through an emphasis on active revision skills. Carving out time for this is not easy, but most teachers find it easy to identify and marginalise some of the "dead wood" in the curriculum. The Primary Strategy already encourages schools to "pick, mix and ignore" when deciding what aspects to cover in detail. So it is important that this approach is properly enshrined in policy so that individual teachers are not left exposed during an inspection.

The DfES is currently encouraging schools to interpret the National Curriculum and the Literacy and Numeracy Strategies with regard to pupil needs, though there is a concern that some OFSTED Inspectors may not be aware of, or perhaps choose to ignore, this development. As ever, the key lies in evidence of success. Provided that there is evidence of an approach being successful the opportunity for improved learning is, I would argue, worth the possible cost of "official" disapproval. Teaching the child must always take priority over covering the curriculum: the often hollow and meaningless "right of access to a broad and balanced curriculum" needs to be weighed against the right of learners to develop functional literacy and numeracy skills. My experience suggests that, once these skills are in place, breadth and balance soon catch up through the spiral nature of the curriculum.

5 STEPS TO A DYSLEXIA FRIENDLY SCHOOL

1. **POLICY** – "Putting practice into policy"
2. **TRAINING** – "Walking the talk "(1)
3. **IDENTIFICATION, ASSESSMENT AND MONITORING** – "Rigorous scrutiny and immediate intervention"
4. **RESPONSES TO NEED** – "Walking the talk" (2)
5. **PARENTS AS PARTNERS** – "Completing the loop"

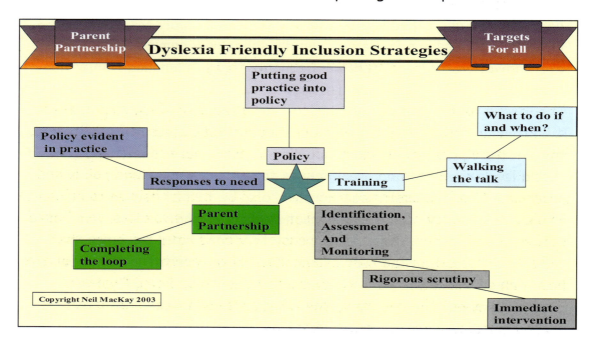

226

1. POLICY - "Putting practice into policy"

Policy is what a school actually does, rather than what is written down in documentation. Therefore many successful schools find that whole school good practice is often ahead of documented policy, and rightly so – someone launches a good idea, the school embraces it and policy will catch up in due course. However the reverse is also true and it can be scary to audit actual practice, write it up as a policy statement and then see if it fits the ethos and aspirations of the school. For example, if a school does not actively require reading materials to be differentiated, it is pursuing a "chalk face" policy of giving children work they cannot read and so is discriminating against weaker readers. While it is very unlikely that this discrimination is enshrined in print, it is policy because it is what is done.

A policy statement will define good practice in relation to Dyslexia and will make it clear to all teachers exactly how this practice is to be delivered, monitored and evaluated. All whole school policies, Teaching and Learning, Monitoring and Assessment etc, will be guided and influenced by the main policy statement and clear guidelines will be available. In consequence a new teacher joining the school will be able to read the documentation and be absolutely clear about the ethos and house style. There is also a strong case for a teacher's monitoring and evaluation at classroom level to be part of performance management, another decision which needs to be implemented at the highest level within the school.

2. TRAINING - "Walking the talk" (1)

The ideal situation is a trained teacher or a teacher in training in every school. This criterion has been fiercely debated because of implications for personnel, resources and funding. However there is a strong view that a Dyslexia Friendly school needs a teacher who can lead policy and practice. Also it is essential that this teacher is in a position to influence whole school policy and ensure that it is translated into classroom based action. The teacher with lead responsibility does not have to be the SENCO unless s/he is already in a position of authority in the school and has been given time to perform this additional role. Being Dyslexia Friendly is about the quality of the 20+ hours each week that a learner spends in mainstream classroom settings.

Unless all teachers know how to make a difference and have their ability to apply their knowledge reviewed as part of performance management, the process is doomed to fail.

Whole school awareness training for all contact staff is essential and schools will be required to keep a log of attendance at training events. A catch up programme will also need to be in place for new staff – teachers and teaching/classroom assistants etc - when they join the school. Evidence will also be required of training needs being identified and addressed on a regular basis. I have been privileged to deliver whole school training in hundreds of schools (First, Primary, Junior, Middle and Secondary) across the UK and it is clear that there is excellent practice in every school. However this excellent practice is not always uniform and may still be dependent upon which teacher the dyslexic learners get.

The challenge of effective training is to identify, validate and celebrate excellent practice while supporting the school to develop "house style" strategies in response to areas of need. Presenting teachers with the issues and asking for deliverable solutions is usually far more effective that any imposition of policy and practice by edict. The School Development/Improvement Plan is also a powerful tool, especially when Dyslexia Friendly initiatives can be linked to other whole school imperatives. For example, there is growing anecdotal evidence that these initiatives are resulting in whole school benefits, including improved attendance, reduced exclusions, improved performance in national assessments (especially by boys) and increased parental confidence.

3. IDENTIFICATION, ASSESSMENT AND MONITORING
– "Rigorous scrutiny and immediate intervention"

There is a need for clearly defined and documented techniques for identifying the unexpected difficulties in acquiring certain skills together with recommended classroom based intervention strategies. "Rigorous scrutiny and immediate intervention" are the watchwords. These perceptive and responsive strategies are part of a school's "anticipatory duty" and are essential if dyslexic learners are to make ability appropriate progress despite current weaknesses in basic skills.

A key attribute of a Dyslexia Friendly school is the willingness to respond quickly to perceived needs without waiting for a formal assessment or "diagnosis" in order to find a label. Making best use of available data will highlight the unexpected problems of a learner who is performing well in some areas but not in others and a speedy classroom based response may be all that is required. When this does not work it can then be topped up by the investment of additional resources, perhaps in the form of School Action and the writing of an IEP.

There is a clear key difference between a traditional SEN approach and the proactive Dyslexia Friendly response. This inclusive, Dyslexia Friendly response comes from class teachers who are empowered to identify learning issues and respond appropriately through reasonable adjustments as part of their commitment to Quality First teaching.

Dyslexia Friendly strategies will need to be evident in everyday marking and assessment, with the link between policy and practice being particularly transparent in this area. For example, many schools have a policy of target marking to highlight a small number of key elements for the learner to address. However scrutiny of books can often reveal that some teachers continue to mark most if not all errors – despite the existence of a policy which states otherwise. This is clearly unacceptable and needs to be addressed through performance management together with training linked to regular monitoring and evaluation. Once again, this type of response needs to be implemented at the highest management level within the school.

4. RESPONSE TO NEED – "Walking the talk" (2)

In a Dyslexia Friendly classroom basic skills which are currently weak, will not be a barrier to ability appropriate achievement. This is a key principle and Dyslexia Friendly schools will be able to show exactly how learners are supported to be the best they can be, even though they may not be able to read it or write it too well just yet. Another important principle is the opportunity for work to be presented and marked in a variety of forms – once again concrete evidence will be available of how policy is to be translated into observable practice. For example, while a paragraph is clear evidence of information processing, so too is a mind map, a story board or a flow chart.

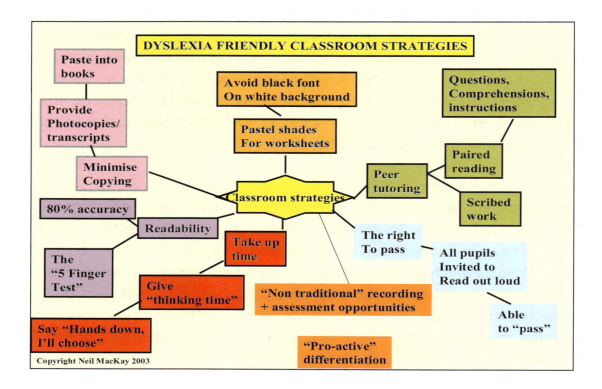

Equally acceptable is information on strips of paper which have been stuck into books. Here a classroom assistant or "study buddy" may have written the information and the dyslexic learner has chosen the order in which it is to be presented. This is a whole school teaching and learning issue which needs to be addressed as part of a coordinated management strategy and built into the school development plan.

Possibly the most controversial principle guiding Dyslexia Friendly schools is the opportunity for discrete, out of class opportunities for small group/1:1 support. This should be seen as a key element of inclusion, which calls for mainstream opportunities without ever stipulating that all of the children must be in all of the classes for all of the time. Thomas Jefferson made the point perfectly when he said:

> *"There is nothing so unfair as the*
> *equal treatment of unequal children."*

In consequence a Dyslexia Friendly school will be committed to the provision of out of classroom opportunities when needs dictate. However there is a concern that schools which do so may find themselves criticised during an inspection for meeting the special needs of a child. It is important to fight against this "one size fits all" approach and to provide evidence that the chosen approach is meeting the current needs of the child. Consider a proud, streetwise 10 year old pupil with currently very weak literacy skills. S/he is likely to need to revisit foundation level skills, perhaps using the sand tray etc, and may be very willing to do so, but not in front of peers in the mainstream classroom. To make a 10 year old work on "5 year old skills" in the classroom is, I would argue, a form of emotional abuse – far better to take the learner out of class and develop the skills with dignity and discretion.

There is a clear balancing act between a child's right of access to the curriculum and the basic skill needs required in order for access to occur. This may result in value judgements being made about the relative merits of certain topics and the need to find more time to reinforce core basic skills. Schools which are committed to teaching the children rather than simply covering the curriculum will instinctively make the right choices and will be able to justify their decisions. These schools are also likely to find that they have very strong parental support for the way learning is organised.

5. PARENTS AS PARTNERS – "Completing the loop"

Dyslexia Friendly schools will enjoy the trust of parents and will be able to provide evidence of this trust in the form of written comments at review, letters of thanks/support and in the way the parents of dyslexic children are involved in the life of the school. A key element in establishing parental trust is the speed with which a school responds to concerns raised and the thoroughness with which dialogue is initiated and maintained.

A frequent question from class/subject teachers is, "How do I respond when parents suggests that their child is dyslexic?" The short answer is that it would have been better if the conversation had been initiated by the school. A problem can occur when a teacher who does not have a specialist qualification in Dyslexia rejects parental concerns with a dismissive "s/he is definitely not dyslexic!" This can be extremely damaging to the child and to relationships with the parent.

A more appropriate response is to acknowledge that Dyslexia might be an issue, to offer to seek further advice and, in the meantime, to agree to teach slightly differently and see if it works. There is an understandable fear that, when a school initiates the discussion, it will automatically require the investment of increasingly rare resources and a worry that it will "open the floodgates". This need not be the case, especially if the standard response is:

- a commitment to teach the child differently in the mainstream setting
- to offer helpful advice for the parents about how to help at home
- to set agreed improvement targets (with parent and child) and to monitor carefully over an agreed period of time
- to report back on an agreed date

If this response does open the floodgates it means that the pressure has been building up for a while – better to deal with it now than wait for an inspection or a series of meetings with angry and frustrated parents.

If this approach works then it is likely that all will be well. However if improvement targets are not met then it is clear that the school needs to take more action, perhaps in the form of directing a teaching assistant to support in class. At the same time the SENCO looks at available assessment data and perhaps does some diagnostic testing. Whether or not a decision is made to make special needs provision and to write an IEP, most parents are happy when the school responds positively to concerns and are willing to suspend their demands for statements and/or statutory assessments if they think that positive action is being taken.

Conclusion

If Dyslexia is accepted as being a specific learning difference it would seem sensible to teach through learning styles and preferences. More and more schools in the UK and beyond are identifying the preferred learning strategies of their pupils and making them the starting point for the preparation of units of work and individual lessons. This inclusive approach has the potential to enhance the learning of all children, from the gifted and talented to those with significant learning difficulties. One benefit of an eclectic learning styles approach is that many apparent learning difficulties may actually turn out to be learning differences which can be minimized or overcome by a change in approach.

Many learners find it difficult to follow complicated instructions, especially those with specific learning differences like Dyslexia, Dyspraxia, Asperger's Syndrome and children with special attention requirements. One response is to develop a whole school commitment to presenting instructions and information in "bite size chunks" and to use positive language.

Target marking, linked closely to lesson aims and objectives, encourages learners and supports the development of their self esteem and emotional intelligence. "Less is more" marking, through the selection of two or three issues to be addressed, is much more manageable and more likely to secure the desired changes. A whole school commitment to the implementation of a target marking policy, together with regular book trawls to assess what is going on, is very Dyslexia Friendly.

The willingness to accept work in different forms is a natural consequence of teaching through learning styles and preferences. It is inclusive to offer choice in the way information is presented for marking because this supports non traditional learners to work with confidence and enthusiasm. End of unit assessments can also be fine tuned to offer choice and learners who have successfully shown what they know through a preferred style seem much more able to revert to more traditional techniques in national exams. From here it is a short step to invest some time in teaching active revision skills so that children know how to learn.

This is particularly important for learners whose working memories are vulnerable. Active revision skills based on their learning preferences can overcome current limitations in working memory and transfer information to the long term memory. Although this approach does take time, it may be a better long term investment than some of the mentoring programmes currently in place to boost "borderline" achievement. It is also much more inclusive as it empowers all children to develop their revision skills, not just a chosen few.

Chapter 16

PUTTING IT ALL TOGETHER
"The opportunities to balance the costs"

Dyslexia Friendly Schools are Effective Schools

They demand excellence from pupils and staff alike and take positive steps to promote staff awareness and competence. Such schools tend to have a zero tolerance of failure and adopt best practice to ensure that all pupils learn. When learning is not happening the schools have the confidence to examine their practice and take action, even at the possible expense of leaving some of the more esoteric elements of the curriculum until very much later, if at all. In my Dyslexia Friendly school "covering the curriculum" is seen as less important than teaching the child. This willingness to place the child's needs at the forefront of curriculum planning leads to flexible approaches to learning.

Dyslexia Friendly Schools are Pro-active Schools

The progress of all pupils is monitored and intervention organized when necessary. Whole school targets are made explicit in the School Development Plan and are supported through carefully targeted INSET to empower teachers to deliver in the classroom. This constant drive to improve achievement of all pupils is reflected in the way assessment and monitoring result in action.

Dyslexia Friendly Schools are Empowering Schools

These are schools in which everyone is important and all pupils are empowered to be the best they can be. A key strategy is the recognition and celebration of individual differences in learning styles.

Dyslexia Friendly Schools are Inclusive Schools

Social, emotional and intellectual inclusion is a top priority in these schools and there is a focus on strengths and abilities rather than weaknesses and problems. Flexible approaches to marking and assessment ensure that currently weak basic skills are not a bar to ability appropriate groupings.

Dyslexia Friendly Schools are Improving "Value Added" Schools

The drive for effectiveness on behalf of all pupils stems from an inclusive and pro-active approach to the identification and fulfilment of all learning needs. This results in pupils who are confident, who understand and believe in their abilities and who are empowered to perform at ever increasing levels of competence.

TAKING IT FORWARD – "More means different"

Most teachers are currently working as hard as they possibly can to meet the demands of the job. However, they are becomingly increasingly worried about children whose needs do not respond to traditional teaching methods. This problem is exacerbated by performance targets which focus on narrowly defined groups of learners and which inevitably marginalize those outside the target boundaries. So the only way that schools and teachers can respond to demands for more is to do things differently, to work smarter rather than harder.

Acknowledging dyslexia to be a learning difference has the potential to motivate and support schools to celebrate diversity and to enhance the achievement of all. Fine tuning of policy and practice is one of the keys to success, a fine tuning which has received the support of teachers across the UK and beyond.

As Dr Harry Chasty used to say:

> *"If they don't learn the way we teach them,*
> *we must teach them the way they learn."*

USING CLASSY WORDS (1)

Noun		Verb

Adjective	Noun		Verb	Adverb

Using Classy Words (2)

The grids above are effective ways of developing the use of adjectives and adverbs. Learners can write in their own choice of nouns and/or verbs, be given a list from which to choose or actually given a grid in which the nouns have been written. The task is as follows:

1. Choose two adjectives to go with each noun
2. Make sure the adjectives fit the words they are describing – try banning words like "big, little and nice"
3. Once an adjective has been used, it cannot be used again
4. Plot the words onto a mind map or flow chart to plan the writing

The task can be given a multi-sensory spin by providing nouns, verbs, adjectives and adverbs on strip of paper to be placed on the grids – this is also a very effective group activity. However it is done, the use of grids can empower learners to write powerful description s in all subjects – it would be a shame to limit this technique to English lessons only.

Precision Teaching

This technique enables teachers and learners to focus on the learning of a small number of words, facts, numbers etc and provides concentrated practice within a short time. It can be used very effectively with tables and number bonds, provided that the amount of new learning is kept to a minimum and is an excellent way of supporting learners to learn jargon words. It works like this:

- Select a manageable number of words or number bonds to be learnt
- Present them over and over again on an A4 page, in random order

---

Precision Teaching in Science

Test tube, beaker, cylinder, chemical, beaker, cylinder, test tube, chemical, cylinder, beaker, ...

- The learner has 60 seconds to read as many words as possible, with the teacher, TA or buddy scoring for right and wrong – this works equally well for spelling, with the words being read out for the learner
- After 60 seconds the learner plots the score on a graph to show the number of words read correctly and incorrectly
- The graph is plotted each time the words are practiced and it is easy to see a developing pattern of increased speed and reduced errors within a very short period of time

The sample below was produced by a primary SENCO to enable a class teacher to provide over learning opportunities whenever the opportunity presented. This is a more ambitious task which reflects the learner's confidence and willingness to accept a challenge.

238

Name: Thomas Dandridge   date:6.2.2003

1.

errors

wispy	crispy	misty	windy	minty	bandy	
softly	coldly	lastly	crisply	limply	costly	
funded	panted	lasted	belted	hunted	wilted	
grasped	linked	limped	jumped	punched	munched	
dampen	crumpet	golden	intent	demist	rafters	
pasta	content	inland	sinking	consent	limping	

2.

wispy	crispy	misty	windy	minty	bandy	
softly	coldly	lastly	crisply	limply	costly	
funded	panted	lasted	belted	hunted	wilted	
grasped	linked	limped	jumped	punched	munched	
dampen	crumpet	golden	intent	demist	rafters	
pasta	content	inland	sinking	consent	limping	

RECOMMENDED READING:

Chinn & Ashcroft   Mathematics for Dyslexics – A Teacher's Handbook   (Whurr)

Dryden & Vos   The Learning Revolution   (Network Continuum Education)

Gardner   Frames of Mind: the theory of multiple intelligences   (Basic Books)

Ginnis   The Teacher's Toolkit   (Crown House Publications)

Given & Reid   Learning Styles – A Guide for Teachers and Parents   (Red Rose Publications)

Hughes   Closing the Learning Gap   (Network Continuum Education)

Hughes & Vass   Strategies for Closing the Learning Gap   (Network Continuum Education)

Knight   NLP at Work   (Nicholas Brealey Publishing)

Ostler & Ward   Advanced Study Skills   (SEN Marketing)

Peer & Reid   Dyslexia: Successful Inclusion in the Secondary School   (David Fulton Publications)

Smith   Accelerated Learning in Practice   (Network Continuum Education)

Riif & Heimburge   How to Reach and Teach all Students in the Inclusive Classroom   (Jossey Bass Wiley)

West   In the Mind's Eye   (Prometheus Books)